REHABILITATION FACILITY
APPROACHES IN
SEVERE DISABILITIES

Publication Number 973

AMERICAN LECTURE SERIES®

A Publication in

The BANNERSTONE DIVISION of
AMERICAN LECTURES IN SOCIAL AND REHABILITATION PSYCHOLOGY

Editors of the Series

JOHN G. CULL, Ph.D.

Director, Regional Counselor Training Program
Department of Rehabilitation Counseling
Virginia Commonwealth University
Fishersville, Virginia

and

RICHARD E. HARDY, Ed.D.

Diplomate in Counseling Psychology (ABPP)
Chairman, Department of Rehabilitation Counseling
Virginia Commonwealth University
Richmond, Virginia

The American Lecture Series in Social and Rehabilitation Psychology offers books which are concerned with man's role in his milieu. Emphasis is placed on how this role can be made more effective in a time of social conflict and a deteriorating physical environment. The books are oriented toward descriptions of what future roles should be and are not concerned exclusively with the delineation and definition of contemporary behavior. Contributors are concerned to a considerable extent with prediction through the use of a functional view of man as opposed to a descriptive, anatomical point of view.

Books in this series are written mainly for the professional practitioner; however, academicians will find them of considerable value in both undergraduate and graduate courses in the helping services.

REHABILITATION FACILITY APPROACHES IN SEVERE DISABILITIES

JOHN G. CULL, Ph.D.

RICHARD E. HARDY, Ed.D.

Diplomate in Counseling Psychology (ABPP)

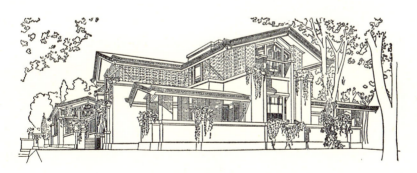

CHARLES C THOMAS • PUBLISHER

Springfield • Illinois • U.S.A.

Published and Distributed Throughout the World by
CHARLES C THOMAS • PUBLISHER
Bannerstone House
301-327 East Lawrence Avenue, Springfield, Illinois, U.S.A.

© 1975, by CHARLES C THOMAS • PUBLISHER
ISBN 0-398-03324-2
Library of Congress Catalog Card Number: 74-16433

Printed in the United States of America
C-1

Library of Congress Cataloging in Publication Data

Cull, John G.
    Rehabilitation facility approaches in severe dis-
abilities.

    (American lecture series, publication no. 973. A
publication in the Bannerstone division of American
lectures in social and rehabilitation psychology)
    Bibliography: p.
    1. Rehabilitation. 2. Handicapped—Psychology.
I. Hardy, Richard E., joint author. II. Title.
[DNLM: 1. Rehabilitation centers—United States.
2. Social service—United States. HD7256.U5 R345]
RD795.C75   362'.0425   74-16433
ISBN 0-398-03324-2

This book is dedicated to three individuals who have made basic contributions to the profession of rehabilitation:

George S. Baroff, Ph.D.
Craig Mills, M.S.
Charles Roberts, L.H.D.

The following are selected titles which have appeared in the Social and Rehabilitation Psychology Series:

CONTRIBUTORS

ROLAND BAXT is Executive Director of Federation Employment and Guidance Service. He received degrees from Brooklyn College and Columbia University. He was formerly Senior Counselor for the National Refugee Service and New York State Employment Service and the Director of Adult Guidance Service. He has been a consultant for numerous assignments for government and voluntary organizations. He is a Board Member, Central Bureau for the Jewish Aged and the Jewish Occupational Council, and member of the Governor's Advisory Council on Developmental Disabilities and the Mayor's Advisory Council on Manpower Planning. Mr. Baxt, a certified psychologist in the State of New York, is a former President of the National Conference of Jewish Communal Service and is active on a state and national level in various Jewish philanthropical organizations related to aging and rehabilitation. He is a Trustee of the New York Personnel and Guidance Association and is a member of the American Psychological Association and the National Rehabilitation Counseling Association. Mr. Baxt has been active with the President's Committee for employment of the handicapped and is a member of the Committee for New York Statewide Planning for Vocational Rehabilitation Services. He has published numerous articles on rehabilitation, educational and vocational guidance, and employment.

A. HOWARD BELL, Ph.D. is Professor of Psychology at Tarkio College, Tarkio, Missouri. Dr. Bell received his B.S. and M.S. degrees from Tulane University in New Orleans and a Ph.D. degree in Clinical Psychology from Louisiana State University in Baton Rouge. Formerly, he was staff clinical psychologist with the Veterans Administration at the V.A. Hospital in Augusta, Georgia and the V.A. Mental Hygiene Clinic in Atlanta, Georgia; he was in private practice and a consultant for the Arkansas Rehabilitation Service in Hot Springs and a consultant for Old Age and Survivor's Insurance; Chief Psychologist and responsible for the development and administration of the Psychology Department at East Louisiana State Hospital in Jackson. Dr. Bell holds membership in numerous psychological associations, is licensed to practice as a psychologist in the states of Arkansas and Louisiana and is certified for practice in Missouri. He has nine other publications and two copyrighted adjustment scales; The Bell Alcoholism Scale of Adjustment (BASA) and The Bell Disability Scale of Adjustment (BDSA).

MILTON COHEN is Executive Director of Federation of the Handicapped, a comprehensive rehabilitation center. Mr. Cohen is Past President of the International Association of Rehabilitation Facilities; Member (appointed by the President) to the original National Policy and Performance Council; Chairman, State Advisory Committee to the New York State Office of Vocational Rehabilitation; Founder and First President of the Metropolitan New York Chapter of the National Rehabilitation Association; Member of the President's Committee on the Employment of the Handicapped; International Consultant to the U.S. Social and Rehabilitation Service; President-Elect of the National Congress on the Rehabilitation of the Homebound and Institutionalized Persons. Mr. Cohen is a leader in working with Congress during the passage of the Javitz-Wagner-O'Day Amendment, revision of the Fair-Labor Standards Act; and revision of the Small Business Administration Act.

JOHN G. CULL, Ph.D. is Professor and Director of the Regional Counselor Training Program, Department of Rehabilitation Counseling, Virginia Commonwealth University, Fishersville, Virginia; Adjunct Professor of Psychology and Education, School of General Studies, University of Virginia, Charlottesville, Virginia; Technical Consultant, Rehabilitation Services Administration, United States Department of Health, Education and Welfare, Washington, D. C.; Editor, *American Lecture Series in Social and Rehabilitation Psychology,* Charles C Thomas, Publisher; Lecturer, Medical Department, Woodrow Wilson Rehabilitation Center. Formerly, Rehabilitation Counselor, Texas Rehabilitation Commission; Director, Division of Research and Program Development, Virginia State Department of Vocational

Rehabilitation. The following are some of the books which Dr. Cull has co-authored and co-edited: *Drug Dependence and Rehabilitation Approaches, Fundamentals of Criminal Behavior and Correctional Systems, Rehabilitation of the Drug Abuser With Delinquent Behavior,* and *Therapeutic Needs of the Family.* Dr. Cull has contributed more than sixty publications to the professional literature in psychology and rehabilitation.

DENNIS A. GAY, Ph.D. is Associate Professor, Department of Social and Rehabilitation Services, University of Northern Colorado, Greeley, Colorado. He received his B.S. degree in Psychology from Oregon State University; M.S. in Counseling from the University of Wisconsin at Madison, and his Ph.D. in Rehabilitation Psychology with a minor in Correctional Administration from the University of Wisconsin, Madison. He was formerly Resident Counselor in an institution for delinquent youth; Vocational Rehabilitation Counselor in an all "Public Offender" caseload serving adults and juveniles, both institutionalized and on parole and probation. Dr. Gay has developed and taught courses in "Rehabilitation of the Public Offender." He has consulted with a number of states on approaches for rehabilitation of the correctional client.

JOAN G. HAMPSON, M.D. received her M.D. degree from Johns Hopkins University, Baltimore, Maryland and she did postgraduate work at the University of Manchester, England. She has held faculty positions at Johns Hopkins and the University of Washington in the departments of Psychiatry and Pediatrics. She has served as a consultant in the Peace Corps, Lighthouse for the Blind and various rehabilitation facilities; she is a Fellow in the American Psychiatric Association. Dr. Hampson is the author of numerous articles concerning sexual precocity and hormonal imbalance.

RICHARD E. HARDY, Ed.D. is a Diplomate in Counseling Psychology (ABPP); Chairman, Department of Rehabilitation Counseling, Virginia Commonwealth University, Richmond, Virginia; Technical Consultant, United States Department of Health, Education and Welfare, Rehabilitation Services Administration, Washington, D. C.; Editor, *American Lecture Series in Social and Rehabilitation Psychology*, Charles C Thomas, Publisher; and Associate Editor, *Journal of Voluntary Action Research*. He was formerly Rehabilitation Counselor in Virginia; Rehabilitation Advisor, Rehabilitation Services Administration, United States Department of Health, Education and Welfare, Washington, D. C.; Chief Psychologist and Supervisor of Professional Training, South Carolina Department of Rehabilitation and member of the South Carolina State Board of Examiners in Psychology. The following are some of the books which Dr. Hardy has co-authored and co-edited: *Drug Dependence and Rehabilitation Approaches, Fundamentals of Criminal Behavior and Correctional Systems, Rehabilitation of the Drug Abuser With Delinquent Behavior,* and *Therapeutic Needs of the Family*. Dr. Hardy has contributed more than sixty publications to the professional literature in psychology and rehabilitation.

ROBERT A. LASSITER, Ph.D. is Associate Professor in Rehabilitation Counseling, Virginia Commonwealth University, Richmond. He has served as Director, Rehabilitation Education and Research Unit, Rehabilitation Counseling Program, and Associate Professor, School of Education, University of North Carolina at Chapel Hill; Technical Consultant to the Rehabilitation Services Administration, Social and Rehabilitation Services, Department of Health, Education and Welfare; Consultant in Continuing Education for the Training and Research Departments, Division of Vocational Rehabilitation in North Carolina and the North Carolina Commission for the Blind; Rehabilitation Counselor, Florida Division of Vocational Rehabilitation; Executive Director, North Carolina Society for Crippled Children and Adults; and State Director, North Carolina Division of Vocational Rehabilitation. His publications include *Vocational Rehabilitation in North Carolina,* School of Education, University of North Carolina, 1970; "Vocational Rehabilitation in Public Schools," *High School Journal,* 1969; "Help for the Mentally Retarded Person," *North Carolina Education Journal,* 1967.

ROBERT J. MATHER is Associate Director, Vocational Guidance and Rehabilitation Services, Cleveland, Ohio. He received his Master's Degree from Kent State University in Rehabilitation Counseling. He is affiliated with the American Personnel and Guidance Association, National Vocational Guidance Association, National Rehabilitation Association and several of the divisions within these organizations. Formerly, he has worked as an Educational Director, Supervising Counselor and Consultant for an independent concern. He has had several publications in the rehabilitation field.

LEON MEENACH is Facility Section Supervisor, Division of Vocational Rehabilitation, Atlanta, Georgia. He was formerly Director of Program Planning and Development, Georgia Office of Rehabilitation Services. Mr. Meenach has served as counselor, supervisor and rehabilitation administrator in the Kentucky Vocational Rehabilitation agency. He has contributed a number of articles in the area of rehabilitation of the psychosocial disabilities and management in a Vocational Rehabilitation agency.

ALFRED P. MILLER is Associate Executive Director, Federation Employment and Guidance Service. He received B.A. and M.A. degrees from New York University. He is President, International Association of Rehabilitation Facilities (New York Chapter); Co-Chairman, Regional Industries for the Handicapped; Consultant and Member of Advisory Committee, Cornell University, School of Industrial and Labor Relations, Rehabilitation Training Program; Chairman, National Legislation Committee for Vocational Rehabilitation, IARF; Chairman, Planning Committee to the Executive of Rehabilitation International USA. Mr. Miller has presented and published numerous articles on vocational rehabilitation. Mr. Miller has been very active in professional affairs.

LEONARD G. PERLMAN, D.Ed. is Associate Executive Director, Epilepsy Foundation of America, Washington, D. C. Dr. Perlman received B.S., M.S., and D.Ed. degrees in Counseling and Psychology from Pennsylvania State University. Formerly, he was Acting Chief in the Training and Education Branch of the National Institute of Mental Health, Division of Narcotic Addiction and Drug Abuse, Washington, D. C. and Supervising

Psychologist at the Work Adjustment Center in Philadelphia, Pennsylvania.

RICHARD N. PEASE, Ph.D. received a B.A. degree from The Rice Institute (now Rice University), Houston, Texas; M.A. degree from University of Kentucky, Lexington, Kentucky and a Ph.D. degree from Temple University, Philadelphia, Pennsylvania. He is actively involved in the private practice of clinical psychology and is a staff clinical psychologist at the Rhode Island Hospital, Providence, Rhode Island. He has a part-time appointment at the University of Rhode Island in Providence. Dr. Pease has had extensive experience in various hospital and psychiatric institutions.

HAROLD RICHTERMAN is Director of the Rehabilitation Services Division, National Industries for the Blind. He received a B.A. Degree from Iowa State Teachers College and a M.A. Degree from New York University in Vocational Counseling. Mr. Richterman has been extensively involved in a number of professional activities related to the rehabilitation of the blind.

HERBERT RUSALEM, Ed.D. is a Professor of Education, Teachers College, Columbia University, and Director of Research and Development, Federation of the Handicapped; Research and Development Consultant to the Mount Carmel Guild, Newark, New Jersey; Quaker Committee on Social Rehabilitation, and National Industries for the Blind; Co-Director of the Learning Capacities Research Project; Author of "Coping with the Unseen Environment"; and Co-Editor of "Vocational Rehabilitation of the Disabled: An Overview." Author of Research Monograph Series on Rehabilitation of Homebound Persons (presenting findings of the Programmatic Research Project on the Rehabilitation of the Homebound).

LOIS OPPER SCHWAB, Ed.D. is Associate Professor of Homemaker Rehabilitation in the Department of Human Development and the Family, Lincoln, Nebraska. Dr. Schwab received her B.S., M.A., and Ed.D. from the University of Nebraska. She has held various positions at the University of Nebraska since

1947. She has been very active in professional affairs relating to homemaking for the disabled, and has received several awards of special recognition including listing in the 8th edition of *Who's Who of American Women*. Dr. Schwab has several publications in rehabilitation oriented journals.

HARRY W. TROOP, M.S. is Deputy Director, Advisory Services and Special Programs, Illinois Division of Vocational Rehabilitation. He was formerly Consultant for Deaf and Hard of Hearing, Chief of Guidance, Training and Placement; Deputy Director, Client Services and Special Programs and Deputy Director, Facilities Planning and Development with the Illinois Division of Vocational Rehabilitation.

JAMES E. TRELA, Ph.D. is Assistant Professor, Department of Sociology, University of Maryland, Baltimore County, Baltimore, Maryland and Research Associate, Vocational Guidance and Rehabilitation Services, Cleveland, Ohio. He received his degrees at American International College, Springfield, Massachusetts and Case Western Reserve University, Cleveland, Ohio. He has done additional post-graduate studies at the University of Washington and the University of Southern California at Los Angeles. Dr. Trela has been very active in research activities in behavioral sciences and sociology and has contributed numerous publications to the professional literature.

PREFACE

REHABILITATION FACILITIES were developed originally to serve blind persons; however, the substantial expansion of the rehabilitation facility movement was centered on developing facilities to serve the mentally retarded. Sheltered work facilities for the mentally retarded sprang up around this country during the decade of the fifties and the sixties. Then as the rehabilitation service model of local services provided through work oriented facilities proved to be so successful persons with other disabilities began being included in this service model. This resulted in the multi-disability facility which we see today.

Expanding and modifying or adapting the service programs in facilities to include clientele with a variety of handicapping conditions has increased substantially the problems of administrators of rehabilitation facilities, but simultaneously this expansion has increased the level and quality of services to all clients. As facilities increased, the spectrum of disabilities with which they worked also increased the skill capacity and working level of the facility. This set of factors result in increased complexity of contract work which the facility can attract.

The purpose of this book is to provide the facility administrator or student of rehabilitation facility administration with an overview of concerns related to serving clients with various disabilities. It is not intended to be exhaustive but is an overview. It is a point of departure.

We are indebted to many who have had an impact on our philosophy of rehabilitation. A few of these significant people include Robert Brocklehurst, Leonarda Crowley, John Parsons, Edward Rose and Joseph Wiggans. We also owe a debt of gratitude to the contributors who worked so diligently to make this book so meaningful to the rehabilitation profession. Special thanks also go to Joanie Mitchell and Libby Wingfield.

JOHN G. CULL

Stuarts Draft, Virginia

RICHARD E. HARDY

CONTENTS

REHABILITATION FACILITY
APPROACHES IN
SEVERE DISABILITIES

PART I

Overview of Facilities

CHAPTER 1

WORKING WITH THE REHABILITATION FACILITY*

THE NEED TO CLARIFY the nature, makeup and value of workshops has long been apparent. There are very few guidelines to help members of the community fully utilize the workshops in their areas. Questions such as: Which clients should or should not be referred to a workshop? What services does a workshop offer? How good is a service of a particular workshop? What responsibility does the workshop have to me? need to be answered. It is the hope of the author that this chapter will supply some of these answers.

One generally accepted definition of a sheltered workshop that has been adopted by the National Association of Sheltered Workshops and Homebound Programs (1966) is as follows: "A sheltered workshop is a work-oriented rehabilitation facility with a controlled working environment and individual vocational goals which utilize work experience and related services for assisting the handicapped person to progress toward normal living and productive vocational status." Within this definition the concepts of "work-oriented rehabilitation facility" and "individual goal" are of prime importance. In the past two decades the sheltered workshop has changed greatly from the early concept of a custodial care institution.

The workshop is now seen as a unique type of rehabilitation agency which affords an individual an opportunity to develop his assets within the framework of a remunerative work setting. Thus, the individual is not only pointing toward competitive employment and a regular, earned wage, but is able to do this within an environment that enables him to experience the digni-

---

* Reprinted from: *Utilization of a Sheltered Workshop* (1969), a publication of a committee of the Workshop Division, Illinois Rehabilitation Association by permission of Mr. Harry W. Troop.

ty and self-respect that comes with being a productive individual.

Types of Workshops

A work activity center is viewed by the Department of Labor and is described in part 25 of the *Federal Register,* July 23, 1968, as a ". . . workshop or physically separated department of a workshop having an identifiable program . . . planned and designed exclusively to provide therapeutic activity for handicapped workers whose physical or mental impairment is so severe as to make their productive capacity inconsequential. . . ." The *Federal Register* goes on to state that this is determined on a basis of whether the average productivity per handicapped worker is less than $850.00 per year. This is measured by dividing the total annual earned income of the work activity center work program less the cost of purchasing materials used; in the case of a work activity center paying at piece rates, the average annual labor rate per client is less than $600.00 as measured by dividing the total annual wages of the client by the average number of clients in the work program.

The term *transitional* reflects emphasis on the development of an individual to a higher level of functioning with the primary emphasis being on moving the person toward employment in the regular labor market. In certain instances, however, the individual may not possess the potential needed to function on a job in a regular labor market; in such instances, the goal may be modified to prepare the person for placement in extended employment (a long-term workshop), additional education, or further supportive services. The transitional workshop is a work setting and not a school, hospital, clinic, or activity center.

Each of the other facilities has distinct programs geared toward meeting the specific needs of the clients. The transitional workshop offers a work experience, an opportunity to identify with the role of a worker (with the resulting dignity that comes from being a productive individual), an environment ideal for evaluation of functioning ability and a setting for work adjustment training (training in self-control, self-discipline, work tolerances, work habits, work performance, work attitudes and knowledge of the world of work itself).

Within a transitional workshop, a client is referred for a specific purpose and for a specific period of time. It is the responsibility of a workshop to document that goals have been established for the client, that they are realistic and that there is movement toward these goals throughout the client's program in the workshop. If the movement toward these goals does not take place, then either the goal has been unrealistic, the workshop has not done everything it can to help that person reach the goal, or the client has reached the point where no more movement is possible. If the goal has been unrealistic, an attempt should be made to correct the goal and bring it within the line of reasonable expectation. If the workshop has not done everything possible, this should be corrected. If the person has reached a plateau and is no longer "moving," the person should be terminated or referred to another more appropriate agency (such as a long-term workshop) if additional movement cannot be forecast within a reasonable period of time.

It is extremely important to keep in mind that there are too few agencies offering services to the handicapped in the community. When a person is maintained in a program longer than is necessary, another individual in that community is, in effect, denied service. If, on the other hand, there is movement but it is slow, consideration should be given to allow this individual additional time to grow at the rate that he is capable. It should not be forgotten that in many cases a person has been disabled all of his life and this has left tremendous damage. These elements cannot be eliminated in a short period of time. Nevertheless, movement toward a goal is essential within a transitional workshop.

Since the goal of a transitional workshop is to develop a person to his highest level of functioning and to move that person out to the regular labor market, emphasis must be on placement. To prepare a person for work but to deny him the opportunity to get a job is folly. Regardless of who does the actual placement, the workshop should have the responsibility either for doing the placement work itself or for following up on the referral to the appropriate agency that will handle the placement activities. Follow-up is a major segment of the workshop program and should not be taken lightly. Too often, people go through a program and are able to function on a job, but since there is no follow-up, the chances of that person maintaining and succeeding on the job are diminished. Much too often minor difficulties arise once the person is out of the workshop, and these difficulties cannot be worked through unless the workshop is in touch with the former client and the employer and has established some system whereby the client feels free to contact the workshop if a difficulty arises. There is no doubt that follow-up services are expensive and quite often handled when "there is time to handle this type of thing." Unless the workshop develops a meaningful follow-up program, much of the value that it accomplishes will be lost in the long run. In keeping with this, it is important for the workshop to include follow-up services in its entire funding process so that it has sufficient funds to handle this very important segment of its program.

The Evaluation and Work Adjustment Center is a highly professional service that falls within the scope of a transitional workshop. Since all transitional workshops make some attempt to evaluate and train clients, transitional workshops that offer evaluation and work adjustment training services must be classified by the type of evaluation and training services they offer.

The long-term, or extended, workshop denotes a continuation of services for individuals who, while in the transitional workshop, have mastered the ability of handling themselves within a sheltered work setting, but upon completion of the transitional program, are unable to meet or to sustain the demands of competitive employment. By moving these individuals into extended employment workshops, they are able to function at their maximum level and are able to achieve success and a level of productivity that is in keeping with their capabilities.

There has been considerable discussion about the advisability of the extended employment workshop being separated from the transitional program when both services are being offered by the same center. The argument that is offered in favor of a separation is based on the desire to provide the person moving into the long-term workshop with a sense of change. Also, it is felt that it is advisable, by the people who argue for a separation, to remove the person who will be functioning in a long-term workshop from the competition and the possibility of not being able to keep up with more competent individuals who are within the transitional workshop program.

The argument in favor of the two programs being together is based on the value of having each group of clients benefit from the stimulation of the other group. While there will always be exceptions to any general rule, most people coming into the transitional workshop may well establish a pattern of competitiveness that would be beneficial for a client in the long-term program. On the other hand, clients in long-term programs will most likely have acquired the discipline, self-control and good work habits that many of the people coming into the transitional program have not yet learned to adopt.

Regardless of whether the two facilities are separated physically, it is important to remember that movement from the transitional to the extended program should not be considered a failure or *terminal* for this disabled person. Many people in industry reach a level of their capacities and spend their working lives at benches, machines or assembly lines. For them, this is terminal employment for which they need not apologize. There should be a similar understanding of the disabled individual who reaches his potential by functioning successfully within a long-term workshop setting.

What is even more important is the need for periodic re-evaluation of the client's place in the extended employment. Disabilities change, human beings continue to grow, the labor market regularly changes, and over a period of time these individuals may be able to move from a sheltered environment into regular employment.

Goals and Objectives of Sheltered Workshops

To ascertain the goals and objectives of a particular workshop, one must examine the stated services offered by the center and then seek clarification of exactly how these services are rendered. It should be clear that not all workshops can offer all services and, indeed, not all workshops should attempt to meet all the needs of all clients. The important thing is that the workshop does, in fact, offer the services it describes in its literature and that the center can show evidence that these services are carried out.

Organizational Structure—Staff

A workshop should have adequate staff to carry out its stated goals. To assess the services that an agency offers, it is necessary to identify who is responsible for each service and how the service is carried out. An example of a basic method of assessing a service, such as counseling, is to find out who does the counseling, what the background of this individual is, how this background prepares this person to provide this service, and how much time during the week this person devotes strictly to counseling.

Programs of Service

Intake

While each workshop will follow its own general procedure for preparing intake reports, it is recommended that a written intake report be prepared after the initial intake interview and that this intake report be sent to the rehabilitation counselor. Items that should be covered in such a report would include the reason for referral, the intake interviewer's impressions of the applicant, the family background, past educational experiences, test material received, medical information, past employment history and vocational goals. The end of the report should include some type of summary that would generally review the material covered in the intake report and would make recommendation as to the acceptability by the workshop of the applicant. If the applicant is an acceptable candidate for the program, suggestions as to services should be written detailing the significant points that the workshop staff should be aware of in dealing with the client, the general goals for the client and how the workshop can go about providing a program that will help the person reach those goals.

Evaluation

In addition to the admission evaluation, which every workshop must offer, there are many types of evaluations that can take place within a facility. The five areas beyond admissions evaluation described below may or may not be offered by any one center; however, the rehabilitation counselor should be aware of what type of specific evaluations can be provided by workshops and where they can obtain the type of evaluation they desire for a particular client.

The purpose of the admissions evaluation is to assess, immediately after a person has entered a workshop, his personal and social characteristics; his present level of functioning; to identify vocational disadvantage(s) (when applicable), and/or limitations; to formulate an appropriate vocational goal and determine the services the individual needs and, if the services are offered, the ability to utilize these services by the individual.

Upon completion of the admissions evaluation, a person in a workshop program must be classified: (1) as not suitable for additional services within the scope of the workshop; (2) as a person who can reasonably be expected to become employable after a program of service, or (3) in need of a longer period of extended evaluation to clarify whether or not he could be reasonably expected to become employable after a program of service.

As mentioned earlier, the workshop is not a medical setting geared to evaluating a person medically. What the workshop can do is to evaluate the client's functioning ability in regard to what he can and cannot do, from a medical point of view.

As a person proceeds through the program, keen attention should be directed to any possible areas of medical limitations which were not originally noted in the medical information. If such evidence does develop, then additional medical consultation is in order. It should be kept in mind at all times that the person is an individual with a specific medical or mental problem and not a diagnostic label without individual identity. Much too often, areas of employment or areas of training are arbitrarily cut off because the person is "an amputee who could not handle such a job." Anyone who has been involved with workshops for even a short period of time will bear witness to the fact that many people can accomplish many things that, on pure medical grounds, are not indicated. While this does not mean that chances should be taken with a person's medical health just to see how far he can go, it does mean that two individuals with the same diagnostic label function in different fashions. The workshop can be a setting to test out a person's functioning and to train him to develop as far as he is capable of developing.

A workshop can offer psychological evaluation, either through its regular staff members or by obtaining these services on a consultative basis. Most likely the evaluation will take place prior to the applicant's entering the workshop. (Rehabilitation counselors customarily refer their clients for psychological evaluation prior to referring them to a workshop.) However, additional testing may be indicated during and at the conclusion of the workshop program, which will assist the staff and the client in planning for the future.

In addition to specific tests, the individual overall functioning within the workshop tells quite a story about a person's makeup. Many times an individual can function at a much higher level than either his IQ or level of academic achievement would suggest. In other instances, a person with an average or better than average IQ score cannot effectively use his potentials and may be, in fact, functioning much less effectively than a person with a significantly lower test score. In addition, a person's ability to handle pressure, deal with supervisors and co-workers, handle failure, peer pressure and a host of other elements related to day-to-day activity of a workshop, may be extremely revealing as to the person's psychological composition.

More and more social and cultural elements loom bigger and bigger as obstacles that hamper the individual's ability to utilize his potentials and to function successfully within the community. Individuals who fall into this category need rehabilitation services just as much as a person with any other type of disability that hampers his ability to function as a productive and useful individual.

A review of the individual's educational experiences may reveal areas of strength, weaknesses, interests, level of academic achievement and potential for additional training. Likewise, his learning ability within the workshop itself will point up significant information as to how he learns best, how well he retains information, whether he can transfer learning and in what areas he exhibits the best potentials.

Within the workshop vocational evaluation takes place as the client is tested in various work situations. Obviously, some workshops will be much more capable of testing people in a variety of work settings than will others. However, most workshops will be able to test people on office assignments (duplicating, collating, stapling, sorting, addressing), quality inspection (visual or mechanical), service functioning (cafeteria work, messenger work, laundry work, maintenance work), bench work (wrapping, packing, assembling), machine operation and, possibly, outside or greenhouse type of work that may be available.

Observation of the client will point up information relating to his ability to follow, retain and carry out directions in a systematic way; capabilities in regard to eye-hand and eye-foot coordination; skills related to depth perception, color blindness and overall visual ability. Also, information can be obtained in regard to the person's physical strength, fatigue level (physical, mental, and emotional) and level of efficiency, organization and consistency of performance. Additional points would include quality and quantity of work under various conditions, personal and social adjustment in regard to co-workers and supervisors, tolerances for routine and monotonous tasks, realistic level of aspiration, level of motivation and drive, habits related to motivation, punctuality and dependability and ability to handle criticism, correction, and a variety of assignments.

Training

The term *work adjustment training* is used to cover a variety of experiences geared toward assisting the person who, by virtue of his handicap, does not possess the attitudes and skills needed to succeed within the regular labor market. Work adjustment training is not trade training. Rather, its goal is to help the individual to develop self-confidence, self-control, work tolerances, ability to handle interpersonal relationships, an understanding of the world of work and a *work personality* that will enable him to handle the day-to-day demands of a work situation in the labor market.

Work conditioning involves numerous items starting with how to punch in on timeclock all the way through to how to handle the receiving of a paycheck in a sophisticated manner. Areas that fall within the scope of work conditioning also include the development of various work tolerances. A few of the work tolerances needed by an employee include the ability to sustain a work effort for a prolonged period of time, the ability to maintain a steady flow of production at an acceptable pace and at an acceptable level of quality, the ability to handle a certain amount of pressure, the ability to get along with all types of co-workers, and the ability to do the unsavory aspects of the job.

It should be remembered that the goal of work conditioning is to help the person to acquire as many skills and tolerances as possible. No one person will necessarily achieve all the tolerances that are desirable; however, in most cases, work conditioning training can result in the individual's being able to function at a level commensurate with his potentials.

Areas that fall within the scope of attitude modification are the development of motivation to work, a desire to give one's best effort to the job at hand, the characteristic of taking pride in what one does, the ability to gain gratification from being productive, the ability to follow the rules and regulations, to do a job one doesn't like, and to accept correction. The desire to maintain as perfect an attendance record as possible, and the acquisition of a sufficiently high level of self-confidence and self-esteem will enable the person to see himself as an individual worthy of respect because of what he can accomplish. When such an attitude is acquired, the person will most likely be able to handle the day-to-day pressures imposed by a job and to handle himself in a mature, self-controlled fashion.

To help the client in learning about the world of work, various techniques can be used such as group meetings, individual counseling, field trips and experiences within the workshop regarding the various areas of the world of work that are discussed or observed in any of the preceding fashions. Emerging from these will be concepts such as: Why do people work? Why does an employer hire a person? What does the employer expect? What should the employee expect? and numerous items concerning earning and spending of money, unions, insurance, vacation, fringe benefits, and taxes. Suffice to say that most individuals within a workshop do not have a good understanding about the world of work and most likely have learned to bluff quite well when asked questions about their knowledge of the work world. By concentrating on helping the person to acquire knowledge about the world of work in a concentrated fashion, the individual can slowly acquire details regarding these matters.

When follow-up takes place for individuals who have been placed by a workshop, a pattern often appears of a person who can make an adjustment to work but who has difficulty handling the personal and social adjustments necessary to function as an independent person. While many of the elements tied into personal and social adjustment should be learned within the home situation, the fact remains that if a person does not achieve this training when he is in the workshop, he may not achieve it at all. In line with this, it is generally felt that some type of personal and social adjustment training is a necessary adjunct to work adjustment training. Areas that fall under the area of personal adjustment training include self-care, grooming and the ability to manage one's life outside a work situation.

A clear distinction should be kept in mind in regard to the difference between vocational training and work adjustment training. Work adjustment training, which has been described earlier, is basically the satisfying of an individual's needs prior to being ready for specific vocational training, i.e. training in auto mechanics or motor winding. In many cases, in dealing with the more severely handicapped person and the mentally retarded, vocational training may not be indicated as much as an entrance type of job that a person may enter after acquiring the skills stressed in work adjustment training. Nevertheless, for an individual who is capable of mastering a particular vocational field that requires specific training, vocational training may well be in order. In certain instances, a workshop may be well equipped to test a person in regard to a specific vocational training. For example, the workshop may well test a person in regard to an interest in clerical work. However, unless they have a specialized department that is geared to prepare people for the clerical field, it may be much more appropriate to refer this individual to a specialized vocational training program dealing with clerical work once the person has mastered the items stressed within the work adjustment program.

On-the-job training is often an ideal type of situation for an individual who may not fit into a specific, formalized program of vocational training, but who can learn the specifics of a particular job outside a workshop. In cases such as these, the employer might be willing to train a person, providing the workshop can establish that the individual has demonstrated the maturity, attitudes and potentials to benefit from a specific program of on-the-job training.

Extended Evaluation

The purpose of an extended evaluation program is to determine whether or not there is a reasonable expectation that additional rehabilitation services might render the client fit to engage in a gainful occupation. It is the rehabilitation counselor's responsibility and prerogative to determine whether or not a client is in need of this type of service.

Under the law, services can be provided within this program for a period up to eighteen months. However, it should be clearly understood that this is the maximum allowable period of time for the establishment of the state agency's third condition of eligibility. During the extended evaluation period, staffings should be held regularly by the workshop and counselor, and justification for remaining in the program should be established. This justification would be derived from reports received from the facility and the staffing sessions that are held prior to the preparation of these reports. It is extremely important that the rehabilitation counselors attend these staffings.

In every workshop there is an admissions evaluation program. This initial evaluation ranges from four to eight weeks depending on the nature of the program and the makeup of the client served. The focus of this initial evaluation is to clarify the individual's level of functioning, appropriate vocational goals, and the services needed to reach these goals. When working with the more severely or multiple-handicapped, it is often virtually impossible to make this determination during the initial evaluation period. Thus, the extended evaluation program provides from up to eighteen months of additional time to determine that there is a reasonable expectation that additional rehabilitation services might render the client fit to engage in a gainful occupation.

The extended evaluation program is not a means to keep a person in a workshop for a prolonged period of time just for the sake of keeping him in the program. The extended evaluation period is for evaluation; however, this does not mean to imply that growth and development do not take place during this time. In fact, considerable training goes on during the evaluation period, and it is this program that brings the person to a point where a judgment can be made as to his future employability. In a case where a person is able to grow and to develop during the extended evaluation program, he can reach a point where it can be reasonably expected that he could be moved on to gainful employment after a period of additional services.

Education

Remedial education may or may not be part of a typical workshop program. Much could be said about the value of offering clients in workshops additional remedial education to help elevate and develop their potentials to make them better equipped to function in the world of work and in the community at large. However, this type of education can often be found in the community, either through regular classroom work or through individual, tutorial work. In workshops that do provide this type of experience, the rehabilitation counselor should give attention to examining the nature of the program and the background of the individual providing this training.

Counseling

Psychiatric counseling is needed when a person's disturbances are rather severe and hamper his ability to function effectively. Obviously, psychotic individuals need psychiatric counseling. Likewise, neurotic individuals and people with other disabling emotional difficulties can benefit from psychiatric services. Quite often in a workshop, psychiatric consultation is available to assist the staff in being better able to understand and work with their clients. In general, this seems to be a very advisable way to utilize psychiatric services and when an individual who is within a workshop program seems to be so disturbed that he does need psychiatric assistance, a referral to an appropriate clinic or therapist is indicated.

Some form of psychological counseling seems indicated when an individual has a handicap that necessitates his being within a workshop program. The trauma of being handicapped, or just being different, handicaps a person much more than one would believe on casual contact. The stigma of not being able to perform at an acceptable level, of always being less than adequate, of never being able to live up to one's own, or to others' expectations leaves a tremendous mark on an individual. Only through some type of psychological counseling, be it intensive or casual, can an individual hope to work through some of his trauma to the point where he can utilize his potentials. In certain instances, this psychological counseling need only be supportive in nature. In other instances, it can become intensive to the point that it verges on services better described under psychiatric counseling.

Vocational counseling is geared toward helping the person establish an appropriate vocational goal and moving toward that goal. Within this area, many issues regarding preparation for employment are covered. Testing can be administered and general guidance provided to help the individual arrive at an appropriate vocational goal.

In most workshop settings, a rehabilitation counselor is responsible for the counseling program of the clients. While emphasis will be placed on helping the client establish and prepare for a realistic vocational goal, many of the points mentioned under the section dealing with psychological counseling become an integral part of what is often labeled "vocational counseling." Effective vocational planning cannot be achieved unless the client enters into some type of counseling relationship.

In addition to providing individual counseling by rehabilitation counselors, a social worker can be extremely valuable as an individual who is able to handle intakes and to work with the client and the client's family. Anyone who has worked within a workshop is well aware of the individual who does not make it because of lack of family cooperation. While getting the families involved with the workshop may be an extremely difficult task, every effort should be made to involve the parents of the client so that everybody is working toward the same goal and so that lines of communication are kept open.

Medical Services

Depending upon the facility, medical services can be a major area of service offered to the client. In workshops that are associated with medical facilities, these medical services can greatly enhance the services that can be offered by the workshop. In cases where medical services are not extensive in nature, the workshop should have access to medical consultation. Prior to entering the workshop, a general medical is obtained by the rehabilitation counselor and, in certain instances, specialized medical information is obtained. This information is important in planning for the program of the client. Much can be said about involving a medical specialist in helping to develop a person's vocational goal in keeping with his medical and physical condition. Likewise, the question of endurance and physical ability to handle a particular goal is extremely valuable. Consultation services or additional, specialized medical evaluation may be indicated as a person proceeds within the workshop program.

Recreational Services

On casual contact with a workshop, recreational services may appear to be a nice addition to a regular program but not necessarily significant in achieving the desired change in the clients. However, as one looks into the background of a typical client in the workshop, it becomes rather apparent that the stigma and deprivation associated with being handicapped affects an individual in many dimensions. One of the major areas in which the person experiences a void is social and recreational experiences associated with the growth patterns of a normal youngster. Clients in the workshop, especially the mentally retarded, are often quite deprived in regard to recreational experiences that are so important in developing coordination, self-confidence, the ability to participate as a team member, physical well-being and a sense of adequacy. Within the workshop, the client acquires a sense of self-worth by being a productive individual. If a person can go beyond this role and acquire the additional sense of being competent within other dimensions of life, such as social or recreational areas, his total growth will be enhanced.

Job Placement

All counselors who deal with workshops are well aware of the time, energy, creativity, and hard work involved in placing a handicapped person in a job situation that is in keeping with that individual's interests and capabilities. While there are a number of resources in the community for securing jobs for handicapped people, e.g. State Employment Service, Vocational Rehabilitation, no one can argue that the more resources a person has in seeking job opportunities, the better the chances of finding an adequate position. In addition, a placement person who is in the employ of a workshop has a much better opportunity to be completely familiar with an individual's assets, liabilities, interests and overall functioning than a placement person in another agency. By being aware of these factors, that placement person can take the time necessary to develop an individualized program of placement, prepare the person for the interview, take the person for the interview and follow-up to see that everything runs smoothly. The workshop cannot expect another agency to take on all these responsibilities and to do them with as much detail and time-consuming effort that a regular staff member in the workshop can.

Follow-Up

Experience indicates that most individuals who complete the workshop program will need some type of supportive assistance during their initial entrance into the job and will have a greater chance of success if they know there is someone to turn to if they run into difficulty, even though they are no longer in the workshop. A placement person or a counselor should be available to the individual when needed. Often, minor difficulties that arise on a job can be cleared up without a great deal of effort by a staff member who is able to provide follow-up services. If this minor event is left unattended, the entire job situation may fall apart. Likewise, the workshop has a responsibility to follow-up, at regular intervals, all people who move out of the workshop in order to insure that they are progressing satisfactorily.

What a Sheltered Workshop Can Accomplish

A sheltered workshop can provide an environment that is conducive to the modification of a client's overall functioning. It can also provide a setting in which an individual can experience success as a productive human being. The makeup of the center can be adapted to meet certain needs of the client through individual programming. A sheltered workshop can develop a work and counseling milieu that enables a person to develop his potentials and to plan realistically for the future.

In certain instances where the workshop is a long-term facility, the center can provide a work situation that enables a person to function effectively even though he does not have the capabilities to handle a job in the regular labor market.

A workshop is not the answer to every client's problems. If an individual is emotionally disturbed to the point that he needs intensive therapy, he will not magically get well in a workshop.

Only when psychiatric services can enable the person to work through his difficulties can he effectively utilize his potentials. Likewise, if a person possesses good work attitudes and basic work disciplines, he may need selective placement, e.g. special trade or academic training, rather than workshop services which are generally geared to the work adjustment approach.

In effect, what must be clarified is the question "What services does a client need and does a workshop specifically provide these needed services?"

Type of Clients to Be Referred to a Sheltered Workshop

In referring a client to a workshop, the counselor should have in mind specific questions that he wants answered. By posing these questions to the workshop, both the staff of the workshop and the counselor can focus on finding answers to the specific elements of the client's makeup that appear to make him unemployable. For example, if a client has had several jobs but has been unable to retain these jobs, the question that can be asked the workshop is "What is the cause of this job failure?" "Has it been that the client has been pushed into jobs that he was unable to handle?" "Is it the client's inability to cope with supervision?" "Is it the client's lack of speed or versatility?" "Does the job lack interest?" "Does the client lack the ability to do things that he doesn't like?"

A counselor may unintentionally view the individual client as a *disability* rather than as a person who has a disability. While the difference may seem subtle, it is quite real when a person is viewed as a *retardate*. Certain generalizations are made about that person that may not be valid. On the other hand, if a person is viewed as an individual who tested out as a retarded individual, then much more emphasis is placed on how the person differs from other people who have a similar disability.

A good example of the need to examine a person as an individual rather than as a disability lies in the generalization often made about retardates being good on boring, repetitious tasks. While it is quite true that many individuals who are retarded do function quite well on repetitious and somewhat boring tasks, it is also quite true that just as many individuals who are retarded become bored and disenchanted with repetitious tasks. One of the nicest statements that has ever been made regarding characteristics of mental retardation is a statement made by a teacher when asked to sum up the characteristics of a retardate. The answer to the question was that, "mentally retarded people are ... people."

In extending this concept of looking at the person as an individual, it becomes quite apparent that while some individuals who are retarded may need a program whereby they can mature, other individuals who have the same label may well be able to move on to a job without a long period of maturation. When people are viewed as individuals and not as disabilities, they are often given an opportunity to try out something; whereas, if all emphasis is placed on a disabling condition, the door might well be closed. This closing of the door is an unfortunate situation. A discussion with any staff member of a workshop will indicate that in many instances a client in the program has greatly outdistanced the original opinion as to how far he could develop and to the extent of growth he could achieve.

What a Counselor Can Expect From a Sheltered Workshop

Workshops have a responsibility to make known to the community the role of the vocational rehabilitation agency and to clarify the nature of their services, misunderstandings and misconceptions about handicapped people. In doing this public relations work, referrals are received by the workshop. These referrals should be referred, in turn, to the vocational rehabilitation agency so that eligibility for services can be determined. The workshop has a responsibility to contact other agencies within the community to make them aware of the type of services the workshop provides and the relationship that the workshop has with the vocational rehabilitation agency.

When a referral comes to a workshop, regardless of how it does come in, an interview should be set up with the intake person to explain the program to the referred person and to establish, as much as possible, the appropriateness of that person's making application to the center. In addition, the individual should be informed of the services offered by the agency and, if the person has not already become a client of the agency, he should be referred to the local office. The intake procedure of a workshop is quite significant and should be done by a professionally competent person. The exact details of what an intake report should contain and how it should be used are described earlier in this chapter.

The workshop should accept the responsibility of handling all necessary intake procedures of referring the client to the vocational rehabilitation agency (if this has not already been done) and of keeping in touch with the vocational rehabilitation agency to ascertain if the applicant is acceptable by VR for sponsorship in the workshop. If the applicant is an acceptable VR client, the workshop should notify the rehabilitation counselor when an opening in a workshop is available and when it could accept that particular client.

Throughout the program, the workshop should keep in contact with the rehabilitation counselor, set up staffings and invite the rehabilitation counselor to such staffings and notify him of any significant changes in the client or his program.

The vocational rehabilitation agency is purchasing a specific program for a specific client. It is the responsibility of the workshop to see that this service is provided and to document that the stated program is, in fact, provided to the referred client.

The workshop has the responsibility of preparing the necessary evaluation reports and of sending copies to the counselor. These reports not only document what has happened to the client, but also point out the nature of the program that will be provided for the next given period of time.

Workshops have been very greatly misunderstood by many people and by other agencies within the community. It is the workshop's responsibility to correct these misunderstandings and to establish a positive program whereby it tells its story to the community and obtains its fair share of recognition and support. By so doing, the needs of the handicapped can be more adequately met and the workshops can achieve more favorable funding support. If the workshop movement is not understood correctly by the people in the community, it is the fault of the workshop; it has not given enough attention to the public relation needs of a service agency.

What the Sheltered Workshop Can Expect from the Rehabilitation Counselor

Attention was given above to methods by which a counselor could assess a given workshop. It is the responsibility of the counselor to follow this process and to become familiar with what the workshop offers and how a counselor might use the services of a workshop for a given client. As mentioned earlier, this can best be achieved by visiting the workshop and meeting with staff personnel. It should be remembered that workshop programs are changing at a very rapid pace and the counselor who may not have had occasion to visit a given workshop for a year or so should, by all means, attempt to revisit and refamiliarize himself with that center.

The rehabilitation counselor has the responsibility to review his client caseload, to assess the possibilities of referring appropriate clients to a given workshop for a given service. In certain instances, it might be very clear that a particular client could be served effectively within a workshop program. In other cases the question of the appropriateness of referral may not be clear. It is in these situations that the rehabilitation counselor should speak with the intake worker of a particular workshop to discuss the appropriateness of a referral.

The rehabilitation counselor should assume responsibility for gathering sufficient case material to evaluate fully the client's handicap, previous contact with other agencies, and present status. Too often, only sketchy material is available on the client and this lack of information hampers the rehabilitation counselor, as well as the workshop intake worker, in accurately ascertaining the client's status and the appropriateness of the referral to the rehabilitation facility.

When it is deemed appropriate for a client to be referred to a workshop and the workshop has agreed that the client is an ap-

propriate applicant, then the rehabilitation counselor should begin processing the case. This involves a medical examination and
psychological testing. In many instances, it may be very necessary to obtain other evaluations to clarify further the appropriateness of the client's being referred and the type of service he
may need in addition to the workshop program. The necessary
authorizations must be sent to the workshop in accord with the
working agreement with the vocational rehabilitation agency. As
the client proceeds through the workshop program, it may become necessary to have additional evaluation or services. It is at
these times that the rehabilitation counselor should discuss with
the staff of the workshop the need for these services and the
most appropriate method of obtaining them.

There is no question but what the rehabilitation counselor's
schedule is quite full and that time to attend meetings at various workshops is demanding. Nevertheless, it is the responsibility
of the rehabilitation counselor to attend and to participate in
these staffings if the client is to receive the best service possible.
By attending and by participating in the staffings, the rehabilitation counselor is kept informed of the program that the person
is receiving and can offer his expertise in developing plans with
the staff of the workshop. If additional services are needed, the
rehabilitation counselor is involved in the initial discussion and
decision making.

One additional fact that should not be taken lightly is that
when a workshop knows that the rehabilitation counselor is truly
involved in the program offered his client, the facility is going
to make a special effort to provide the best program possible and
to work closely with the counselor. Few things stimulate workshop staff more than having outside people ask questions. Often,
the workshop may be so wrapped up in its own program that it
has difficulty seeing things from an outside perspective. The rehabilitation counselor, by asking these questions, can provide
this stimulation.

The report that the workshop sends to the counselor should be
reviewed and, when necessary, clarified by asking questions. Too
often, reports are briefly scanned without giving attention to the

details that tell the total story. Thus, a clear picture is often not obtained and the client may well suffer.

Each workshop has an agreement with the vocational rehabilitation agency which spells out in detail the exact relationship between the center and the agency. By being familiar with this agreement, the counselor is aware of what services the workshop offers, how these services are provided and what he can expect from the center. From the workshop's point of view, by having the counselor familiar with the working agreement, there is less chance for misunderstandings and confusion.

The rehabilitation counselor has the responsibility to be familiar with workshops and their operation. This can be accomplished by becoming familiar with the working agreement between the state agency and workshops in his area, by exchanging information with workshop staff members, by attending professional meetings, and by keeping up on professional literature regarding the field. With this type of information, the rehabilitation counselor can better utilize the facilities in his area and can make a contribution to the overall movement of workshops in general.

In the preceding sections, an attempt has been made to describe the responsibilities of the workshop and of the vocational rehabilitation agency. In reference to mutual responsibilities, the most significant element is to work together as a team. A workshop's only purpose for existence is to provide meaningful programming for handicapped individuals. The state agency's only purpose for existence is to provide services to these same handicapped individuals. Much too often communication breaks down between agencies and misunderstandings can develop. Both the workshop and the rehabilitation counselors have a responsibility to maintain close and open communication, to raise issues that are not clear and to resolve these issues as they occur. By maintaining this type of cooperative arrangement, the client obtains the best possible services as quickly and as effectively as possible.

PART II

Working With the Socially and Emotionally Disturbed

Chapter 2

SERVING THE EMOTIONALLY DISTURBED IN REHABILITATION FACILITIES

Richard N. Pease

Introduction

THE MAIN PURPOSE of this chapter is to acquaint the newly appointed rehabilitation facility administrator and rehabilitation administration student to some of the practical problems associated with employment in the mental health field. The emphasis and perspective presented contains a bias of the clinical practitioner, without the usual academic-research orientation of most introductory textbooks. Some ideas that are presented in this chapter are personal and opinionated. They are shaped by the author's experiences as a clinical psychologist who is actively engaged in clinical work in the mental health field on a daily, full-time basis. However, this is balanced by an attempt to objectively assess the current status or state of affairs within the mental health field by reflecting trends and viewpoints of other experts known to the author personally or whose works the author has read within the past several years. Every effort has been made to make this presentation current and up-to-date.

The vastness of the mental health spectrum with respect to problems in living, types of facilities, treatment methods, personnel, and administrative problems, preclude more than an introduction and overview. Furthermore, the approach in this presentation is designed to give the newly appointed mental health administrator and student more of a feel for the mental health field in its practical aspects. An assumption is made that the reader comes to this chapter already prepared with some basic knowledge about mental and emotional disturbances and the general field of mental health. The following sections will deal with topics such as the history of Western civilization's treatment of disturbed behavior, types of mental disorders, types of

31

treatment facilities, large state-operated hospital institution facilities, expectations and pitfalls for the new administrator, and conclusions in the summary, condensed form, emphasizing practical implications.

History of Western Civilization's Treatment
of Disturbed Behavior

From the beginning of recorded history problems in living have existed in terms of survival, the relating of one person or group of persons to another individual or group, and man's relating to his physical environment. The theory of evolution backed by evidence from many disciplines such as archeology, anthropology, and paleontology provides a basis for speculating about the plight of early humans on this earth with regard to life demands, problems in living, and how various groups adjusted to the stresses of their existence. We are concerned with this type of speculation only to establish an assumption that at least within the immediate history of mankind dating back 40,000 years or more, human nature has probably not appreciably changed from a biological point of view. People living today are probably not physically unlike people who lived 1,000, 2,000, 10,000, or more years ago.

Throughout the more recent recorded history of Western civilization, such as in the Old Testament of the Bible, there is ample reference to mental and emotional problems which are not unlike those observed today. At various periods in this history, diversified attitudes and beliefs evolved regarding disordered behavior as to its cause, course, and treatment. Well documented examples of thought disorders, disturbances of mood, organic brain dysfunctioning, antisocial behavior, and mental retardation dot this particular time in the history of Western civilization.

The prevailing beliefs of any specific time period and the status of knowledge regarding disturbed behavior shaped the treatment techniques toward those individuals that became afflicted. Thus, we read in history books of people in the past being possessed by demons, evil spirits, and witches, who were socially ostracized and treated with fear and contempt. Exorcisms and such cruel methods of blood-letting, drilling holes in the skull (trepanning), beatings, and torture, often until death, flourished through the ages right up until the eighteenth and nineteenth centuries. Changes were brought about by the reforms of Philippe Pinel and similar counterparts in the U. S., such as Dorothea Dix and Clifford Beers, that have extended into the twentieth century (Coleman and Broen, 1972).

There were notable exceptions to this such as the moral therapy movement of the first half of the nineteenth century from 1800-1850 (Bockoven, 1956; Taulbee and Wright, 1971). Many of the mentally disturbed of that time were treated with kindness, understanding, support, and helped to recover their capacity for self-sufficiency and work. Unfortunately, this movement ended with the onset of an evolving medical model and the coinciding of the development of large institutions for the mentally ill. The reforms that brought an end to some of the cruel, inhumane treatment were followed by great hopes for physical cures that never materialized. These hopes still persist with much active research going on at present in attempts to find a physical, neurochemical, or genetic cause for perplexing disorders such as schizophrenia, manic depressive psychosis, and psychotic depression.

Although there were other exceptions in history of humane treatment and enlightened views of disordered behavior, the overall picture in the Western world was generally bleak for a person who developed any severe psychological problem in living. These individuals had to solve their own difficulties or were at the mercy of, hopefully, sympathetic family and friends. They were usually ignored or treated with one of the methods described above. If the person responded favorably, the efficacy of the method employed was reinforced. On the other hand, if the response was unfavorable, often greater pressure was utilized before the person was abandoned as hopeless and beyond help. At this point in time, the consequences of being a lifelong outcast, imprisoned, or put to death were very real.

Syphilis had been a major factor in the large number of admissions to mental hospitals and institutions in the late 1800's and early 1900's. Many of these patients exhibited progressive mental deterioration known as general paresis of the insane. With the discovery of the cause of syphilis in the late 1800's and early 1900's, there was hope for breakthroughs for other forms of disordered behavior through medical and biological research (Coleman and Broen, 1972). When this did not occur, a sense of hopelessness and abandonment grew. Large institutions for the mentally ill became dumping grounds for many unfortunate people. Chronic institutionalized life styles were common with people living out their lives at a state institution or hospital. These large facilities became total communities, self-sufficient in many respects with their own dairy and truck farms, laundries, kitchens, hospitals, and maintenance departments. Much of the labor was performed by patients who were either paid nothing or a minimal salary, but provided them with an escape from the routine of boredom and inactivity.

While this life style of institutionalized living was far from ideal since many abuses resulted in such settings, for many patients these facilities became havens from the outside world and its overwhelming pressures. They provided a community where one could have his/her basic life requirements taken care of, engage in simple work, and pursue other recreational activities. For the families of these patients and for society, placement in such institutions frequently resolved everyone's *problems.* Shame, embarrassment, fear, and problems of responsibility of families and patients alike contributed to this deplorable situation. Few voices have been heard in protest and, by and large, public apathy reigns even today. Conditions have gradually deteriorated further as less money has been invested by the public; buildings have been poorly maintained, morale problems among employees, and attitudes of custodial care and hopelessness pervade the scene right up to the present day.

Of course, there were some exceptions at various hospitals and there were individuals who worked hard and who were dedicated against increasing odds (Shakow, 1969). Without hope it was difficult to attract professional personnel such as psychiatrists, psychologists (few in the early 1900's), social workers, and nurses, because they often sought positions in private sanitoriums, community hospitals, and in private practice. This recruitment problem exists in many of today's state institutions and public hospitals; this problem will be discussed more fully later in this chapter.

Over the past seventy years treatment techniques have come into vogue, resulting in high hopes for a breakthrough. In most cases these techniques were overused, then found to be less effective than first presented. In time they were either abandoned or refined clinically for selected cases and specific problems. Prominent examples can be seen in the eugenics movement at the beginning of the twentieth century with widespread emphasis on genetic causes, resulting in sterility laws and sterilization. Other examples are seen in psychosurgery, insulin shock treatment, and electroshock treatment therapies of the 1930's and 1940's. Insulin shock treatment has now been largely abandoned in the United States. Electroshock treatment has been refined and is now used primarily for selected cases of severe depression, especially in the middle years of life, and for some acute schizophrenic reactions. Psychosurgery has more recently been given a new life with refinements in techniques for pinpointing and destroying brain tissue resulting in some successes in selected cases of epilepsy and Parkinson's Disease. The archaic methods of destroying large areas of brain tissue that occurred in lobotomies and lobectomies have been abandoned.

The most recent example of this over optimistic hope for a breakthrough still continues in the use of chemotherapeutic agents. In the early 1950's tranquilizing drugs were first introduced on a large scale and hope for emptying the state hospitals and other institutions ran high. But like previous treatment approaches, these hopes have not been fully realized. Although many patients were helped and management became easier, waves of discharged were often followed by gradual readmissions. The use of drugs has now become more specialized with attempts to match particular disturbances with specific drugs or combination of drugs at effective drug dosage levels. Research continues to expand in the drug field at a tremendous rate, while on a practical level, drugs are administered on a clinical basis, often reflecting the individual doctor's clinical experience rather than any proven effectiveness of the prescribed drugs. With this brief historical background, our attention will now focus upon types of disorders, facilities, and treatment methods.

Types of Disorders

The basic types of mental, emotional, and behavioral disorders have probably remained relatively unchanged over the years, although the symptomatic manifestations have been influenced by cultural and social changes. A few notable exceptions, however, are with disorders such as general paresis of the insane, which has declined with the diagnosis, treatment, and understanding of syphilis (Coleman and Broen, 1972). Another exception on a more negative side is the current product of the drug revolution of the 1960's that has produced large numbers of multiple drug users in the teenage, adolescent, and young adult age groups. In the present day because of the widespread availability and usage of drugs, there are also more persons seeking help whose basic problems in living are further complicated by drug usage.

For practical purposes and expediency the population of mentally disturbed can be roughly divided into four major groups. The first is a severely incapacitated psychotic group.* These persons usually need some, or at least, temporary hospitalization and medical treatment. With appropriate medication and adequate psychological treatment, many of these acutely disturbed people can now be treated on a short-term basis in a hospital setting, then discharged to an outpatient status for more intensive, long-term, or supportive treatment and follow-up. For those who are not able to be treated within a few days up to two or three weeks, more extended hospitalization may be necessary, but rarely beyond several months. When this type of patient is discharged, a return to the community is generally advisable and

---

* For a fuller account of mental disorders the reader should consult the Diagnostic Manual of Mental Disorders (see reference) and a basic textbook in abnormal psychology such as Coleman and Broen, 1972 (see reference).

can be accomplished. Halfway houses, group homes, and other semi-protected facilities may help to bridge the gap back to the community for the most incapacitated cases.

The second large grouping consists of psychoneurotic and psychophysiological reactions. These people rarely need hospitalization except for diagnostic work-ups, situational crises, threats of suicide, or for complicating physical reasons. Most of these people can be treated as private patients of physicians, referred to a mental health clinic, or to a private practitioner in psychiatry, clinical psychology, or psychiatric social work. If hospitalization is necessary, a general hospital with a psychiatric unit often meets this need very well. In some cases such people may go to a longer-stay facility such as a private mental hospital or sanitorium depending on financial resources and/or third party hospitalization coverage.

A third major group is the addictive disorders. Although alcoholic problems have much in common with other forms of drug addiction, traditionally the alcoholic has been treated either in a general medical facility or in a separate program specifically designed for alcoholics. This state of affairs still exists since many alcoholics are seen for acute problems through the emergency departments of most general hospitals, where they are often discharged without a follow-up treatment program beyond recommendations to see their private physicians, or they are told to go to AA. Within the inpatient population of any large general hospital there are *hidden* alcoholics who are treated for secondary physical problems without being labeled or diagnosed as having an alcoholic problem. Chief problems in these latter cases include various gastrointestinal, digestive tract disorders, such as ulcers, pancreatitis, and liver dysfunctioning. Because of the acute need to diagnose and treat these physical difficulties, the primary underlying disorder of alcoholism may be overlooked or dismissed. The alcoholic and his/her family contributes by keeping the problem hidden in many cases. There is also a reluctance to diagnose or deal with alcoholism by hospital and private physicians because of the lack of expertise to treat these disorders as well as the poor prognosis and time involved.

When the alcoholic problem is appropriately recognized and

diagnosed, treatment generally entails a referral to a local AA branch or to a state alcoholic bureau or treatment center. Some of the more affluent and educated may seek out treatment with their family doctor or a psychiatrist for private psychotherapy. When there are serious complicating physical factors, the best outpatient treatment may involve a multidiscipline approach with an internist handling the physical problems, a psychiatrist or other skilled mental health worker concentrating on the psychosocial aspects of the drinking problem, and often supportive assistance through the various self-help programs such as AA and Al-Anon. Of course, before a treatment program of this variety can be fully implemented, especially in the more serious, heavy drinking cases, hospitalization may be required to detoxify and withdraw the person from alcohol, to improve the patient's physical health, and to treat any other acute physical problems.

With regard to other drug addiction problems, such as physically addicting cases of heroin, cocaine, and morphine dependency, similar problems exist. Often these persons do not seek help voluntarily or directly for their drug habits, except in crisis situations involving withdrawal, arrest, or physical illness. Because of the high costs of maintaining such habits, most of these addicts must resort to stealing, shoplifting, prostitution, and selling drugs themselves, making them vulnerable to arrest and incarceration. The courts often give these addicts the choice of prison or entering a drug treatment center. These centers are mainly self-help settings manned by ex-drug addicts and modeled after Synanon and Daytop. Treatment is long-term; the usual stay is eighteen months to two years plus follow-up involvement with the program. The dropout rate is extremely high as many addicts choose treatment mainly to avoid prison sentences but then leave the program at the first opportunity to return to the streets or to a similar drug culture in another city or state. The treatment program in these residential treatment centers focus on group encounters, confrontations, and marathon sessions designed to break down the addict's rationalizations and his attempts to *con* other people, while trying to build greater self-confidence, responsibility, relationships with others, and independence.

With the drug revolution of the mid 1960's to early 1970's, such centers and programs have spread across the country. In addition to these resident programs there are drop-in, drug information, and counseling centers, and drug programs associated with existing facilities in general hospitals, psychiatric hospitals, and mental health clinics. With the increase in drug experimentation, availability of many kinds of drugs, and a widespread usage across the socioeconomic scale, there are now more cases of multiple drug usage without physical addiction. There are many more cases of *soft* drug dependency involving marijuana, amphetamines, and barbiturates. There seems to be a decline in the use of some of the hallucinogenic agents, especially LSD, probably because of the reports of possible genetic damage.

There also appears to be a trend toward combining alcohol with soft drugs. This trend may be partially reactive to greater efforts in the enforcement of drug traffic laws and the lowering of the legal drinking age from twenty-one to eighteen in most states. Beer and sweet wines have begun to replace some of the illegal drugs. The liquor industry has anticipated this and has responded to this trend by increased production and advertisement of pop wines and beer, which focus on the younger generation. There has also been increased promotion of the smoother, lighter Canadian-type blends of whiskey and bourbon for this same reason.

Mention should be made in this context of other important addictive, health-impairing problems that are often not included in the usual mental health caseload. Specifically, cigarette smoking and overeating problems abound in our culture (Bruch, 1973; Mayer, 1968). Although there are various efforts to educate the public, such as through the American Cancer Society, American Heart Association, and the National TB Association, little treatment is available except through private practitioners and self-help groups. There are some specific clinics in general hospitals for obesity problems. In the self-help type group,

Weight Watchers represents the best known organization which has spawned other groups such as Overweight Anonymous. The mental health agencies should pay more attention to these problems which represent major health hazards to large portions of our population.

The last major group to be considered is the aged and problems of organic brain dysfunctioning associated with the aging process. This group is increasing as the general population grows older and many people are forced to retire at early ages. Various disorders of circulation, such as arteriosclerosis and atherosclerosis increase with age, creating problems of mentation with resultant effects on personality functioning. The shifting patterns of family life with a general breakdown of the extended family cohesiveness has given rise to emphasis on the smaller nuclear family unit, which has created additional problems for the elderly. All of these factors have contributed to taking away their support, usefulness, and have created loneliness and alienation for a large number of the elderly. For many of them the stresses of living overtax an already faltering mental functioning and declining physical capacity resulting in various psychological disorders of the aging.

The more difficult to manage and regressed aging patient, especially with poor financial resources, often ends up in a geriatric ward or unit at the state hospital or in a nursing home setting supported by Medicare and other public funds. An atmosphere of hopelessness and helplessness pervades many of these facilities, almost completely negating any positive response to treatment. For some there is a resignation to impending death, which may well be hastened by a lack of will or purpose to continue living combined with often minimal, if not inferior, medical and nursing attention. With proper medical attention, nursing care, and general supportive care, many of these psychiatric casualties can and do improve, some to a point where at least a sense of human dignity is restored and in other cases even a return to some level of productive living. Improved aftercare facilities certainly would be necessary to expend these efforts, such as creating more group living situations, halfway-type houses, and other supportive living arrangements. With more direct aid and treatment, many elderly could remain at home and in the community without hospitalization or after brief hospitalization for diagnosis and treatment of acute physical and emotional problems.

Beyond these major groups of disorders, there are many other problems which could be discussed to make this presentation complete, such as sexual disorders, social dysfunction, personality problems, mental retardation, and transient situational disturbances, not to mention the whole field of child learning and behavioral disorders. The handling of all of these problems is similar to some of the above groups, based upon availability of services, the severity of social and personal dysfunctioning, and the general requirements for treatment. The reader should consult other references for more specific information about any specific disorder or type of problem (Coleman and Broen, 1972).

Types of Treatment Facilities

Our discussion will concentrate on facilities serving the adult, although many of these facilities also provide services to children. Children present somewhat different problems and treatment approaches, specialized facilities, and programs, especially with regard to educational difficulties and severe acting out behavior disorders. Therefore, in this section we will not discuss such child treatment areas as special education classes for the emotionally disturbed child, child guidance-type agencies, child residential treatment facilities, programs for the emotionally disturbed child, and other pediatric mental health services designed specifically for the treatment and/or prevention of behavior and emotional problems in children.

To a great extent the type of client seen in a mental health setting will be determined largely by that treatment facility, its staff, philosophy, approaches, geographical location, referral sources, and the needs of the general population who will use that facility and service. To classify current treatment facilities is very difficult because of such diversity. There are many changes as old facilities take on new directions and new agencies spring up to meet some pressing current need. Looking over the whole spectrum we can identify types, describe and comment upon some of the major existing facilities and services currently available throughout the United States.

First, the private practitioner or member of the clergy represents the professionals most likely to encounter individuals in distress and personal conflict. The American Medical Association and the medical profession have been very successful in convincing most people that if they have a problem, the family doctor is the first one to consult. Religious leaders have also served in similar roles providing counsel to their parishioners about problems in living, whether or not moral or ethical issues are involved. Consequently, priests, ministers, and rabbis have often been the first to be consulted by many people in trouble.

While the private physician and religious leader has continued to be the initial contact for many individuals with mental health problems, more recent trends are toward other professions and agencies. Thus, mental health clinics, hospital-based clinics, clinical psychologists in private practice, social workers, marriage counselors, and a variety of self-help and specialized resources such as drug problems, suicide prevention centers, crisis intervention clinics, and neighborhood health centers have become resources to turn to in times of personal stress.

Oftentimes mental, emotional, and personality difficulties produce secondary physiological and physical symptomatology, which propels a person to go to his family doctor, internist, or to a medical specialist dealing with the particular symptom. For example, a person with a gastrointestinal symptom may go to an internist or gastroenterologist, and a person with a urinary symptom may consult an internist or urologist. Unfortunately, many of these well-trained, competent, medical specialists, as well as many general practitioners, fail to identify such symptoms as psychological. Thus, they treat them inadequately, usually with pat instructions that the patient cannot follow, such as "relax" and "don't worry." Medication is often prescribed for the symptoms without appropriate follow-up of its effectiveness. Many times the problem is simply dismissed as unimportant if no physical cause can be found. In the latter situation the patient may be told that there is nothing wrong physically and that it is *emotional* or *nerves* but without any real explanations or treatment plan. Nevertheless, many people improve under these conditions, primarily because of benefits associated with reassurance that there is no health-threatening disease present, the support of the doctor-authority figure, suggestion, use of tranquilizers, benefits of ventilating worries and concerns to another person, and merely the passage of time which enables most people to live through a brief life crisis.

The above description is generalized, but nevertheless it points to some glaring problems in handling mental health complaints. The average physician, excepting the psychiatrist, is generally not prepared by education or training to adequately diagnose or treat mental and emotional disorders. This problem is further compounded by the element of time that may be involved. Unlike most physical disorders and diseases, mental health problems require considerable time to investigate diagnostically and even more time to treat. The medical-biological orientation of many physicians, as well as the real problems of time and the number of patients in need of help, prevent even the most competent medical man from giving adequate treatment. Even where supportive help and/or chemotherapy are the best treatment approaches, most medical men tend to under-prescribe medication because they have not developed the clinical experience with certain drugs used by the psychiatrist. Thus, many times the dosage of a tranquilizer or antidepressant is so low as to be ineffective or palliative at best. Without adequate follow-up, there is no way of gauging the drug's effectiveness or whether the patient is actually following through as the doctor directed. The problem of self-medication is a very common and a real problem. All of us in the mental health field frequently see people who tell us about taking Valium® or Librium® whenever they feel nervous or cannot sleep. The only time that these people return to their original physician who prescribed the drug is when the prescription has expired or because of some side effect.

The above situation is generalized to illustrate some major

problems in this area. There are many physicians who have developed, often on their own initiative, the expertise to diagnose mental health problems. They recognize the importance of these problems and seek other expert consultation, refer them to appropriate treatment facilities or to other mental health specialists such as psychiatrists, clinical psychologists, and psychiatric social workers. The younger, more recently trained physician, especially from the United States medical schools, is generally more sophisticated and better trained in the diagnosis and treatment of mental health problems than his predecessors. More medical schools, intern, and residency programs have recognized this area and have incorporated courses, appropriate experiences, and training regarding mental health problems.

The religious leader is another key individual in the mental health field who encounters some of the same problems that the physician does, especially with regard to expertise and training. Time generally is not as great a problem for the religious leader who may see individuals and groups for as long as other professionals in the mental health field. More critical are issues of training, expertise, and relevance. As is true with the younger physicians, priests, ministers, and rabbis are now better trained to cope with mental health problems than their predecessors. This correlates with an increased social awareness and social action movement that has developed in our country and around the world in recent years and has affected the religious communities profoundly.

However, the problem of relevance remains an issue in terms of attitude and orientation for the religious leader in approaching people with problems in living. Many people are "turned off" when their distress is translated into ethical-moral terms and given pat answers such as to "pray more," and "not show despair." A person confronted with an acute problem of, say, a dissolving marriage or a deepening depression, may sometimes be thrown into a more perilous conflict because of their specific religious leader's position regarding alternatives. An objective, nonevaluative, yet supportive approach may be extremely difficult for a religious leader without extensive training and personal maturity. He may find himself in a conflict to remain true to his religion and at the same time to be an effective psychotherapeutic agent.

A plethora of group services have developed because of the increasing demand for mental health services which has come about because of corresponding improvement in education, with more sophisticated awareness of such problems, with a reduction in the social and personal stigma associated with such services. The third revolution in mental health has come about with the community mental health movement emphasizing diagnosis and treatment on an out-patient basis close to the person's residence (Goldenberg, 1973).

Primary in this community mental health movement has been the establishment of community mental health centers across the United States, subsidized heavily by the federal government with matching state monies. Most of these centers have been established with a traditional outpatient clinic structure, involving a mental health team of psychiatrists, clinical psychologists, and psychiatric social workers. There was originally considerable disagreement of professional territory in the earlier mental health clinic efforts regarding administrative control of many of these centers. The medical profession had the control traditionally, and, of course, wanted to continue to retain this position. However, economics dictated the scene since few psychiatrists were available on a full-time basis to administer a center at salaries that could be afforded. Consequently, the clinical psychologists and psychiatric social workers, relatively few of whom were in their own private practices, moved into these administrative posts. In fact, because of economies, more and more administrative positions are now being filled by social workers as more clinical psychologists have entered into private practice. A truce or compromise of sorts has evolved with a psychiatrist, often part-time, maintaining medical control while administrative functions are performed by an executive director, usually a social worker or clinical psychologist. Perhaps, the next step will be in having professional administrators, as the psychologists and social workers find other positions more lucrative and/or more satisfying. Of course, this would make perfectly good sense as neither the average psychiatrist, clinical psychologist, nor psychiatric social worker is qualified by training or expertise to function in an administrative position. As greater accountability for quality service that must meet good cost-efficiency standards, especially with more third party reimbursement, the need for specially trained mental health administrators should increase.

The community mental health clinics have not as yet fulfilled these high expectations that were envisioned several years ago. The problem seems to be one of number of patients as well as outdated diagnostic and treatment approaches. As their services became known to the community, many of the centers were inundated as soon as they opened their doors. This simply reflects the fact that more people avail themselves of services when they are readily available at reduced fees on a sliding scale than they would to private treatment. The stigma has declined somewhat, especially with more public education that emphasizes that treatment is needed for mental illness as is needed for physical illness.

The problems of approach and orientation are also important. Too many mental health centers have unwittingly adopted the old child guidance clinic model and format. For example, new clients are seen for intake by the social worker and then referred for further diagnostic assessment to the psychiatrist and/or clinical psychologist. Following this workup, the client's case is presented at a team conference and a treatment plan is devised with the client being finally referred back to one of the team for treatment. Follow-up treatment is handled usually by the clinical psychologist and/or psychiatric social worker, although the psychiatrist may see some clients for psychotherapy, to review medication, or for consultation if alternative treatment such as hospitalization becomes necessary. All of this diagnostic work takes precious time, a luxury that cannot be afforded when such large numbers of people need help.

Too much traditional individual treatment is practiced compared to shorter, limited goal directed treatment and use of group and family procedures. Innovative techniques and newer approaches have entered into the treatment armamentarium, but at a slow pace, often without administrative direction. For example, individual workers may decide to use some techniques he/she finds useful, while co-workers continue to use traditional approaches for the same types of problems without concern as to appropriateness and/or expense in time and personnel. There is a definite need for administrators to keep pace with changing times, review the agency's philosophy of treatment, its mission, and to work toward more effective, shorter treatment approaches that will better serve the needs of the center's client populace. The use of lesser trained personnel with appropriate training and consultation provided by the "experts" should be pursued further. The arithmetic is simple enough as there will never be enough psychiatrists, Ph.D.-level clinical psychologists, and certified master's level psychiatric social workers to meet the demands for mental health services in our society at the present rate of training. While we may look to our training institutions with an aim of turning out more specialists at a faster rate, the economics and time reveal that this is not a viable solution.

Many people have reached this last conclusion a long time ago and there has been much discussion about training and using "lay workers" in the mental health field (Joint Commission, 1961). However, putting this concept into actual practice has been slow and sporadic. The professionals have not led the battle very aggressively, and can be accused at times of protectiveness and/or indifference as they busily pursue their own jobs, ignoring the larger issues confronting society. Like so many social problems, the demand will often dictate the solution, not waiting for the expert-professionals to lead the way.

This is exactly what has occurred with many self-help types of services that have emerged in recent years. A primary example is the drug prevention and rehabilitation programs that sprung up to meet the public's alarm as drug abuse spread across the socio-economic scale in the mid-sixties to early seventies. Prior to that time treatment of drug addicts was confined to several large narcotic hospital-prison complexes, a few self-help programs like Synanon, and individualized efforts at general hospitals, private hospitals, and existing state institutions with a few addicts receiving private treatment. Even then the success of the professional was low. Many professionals today continue to assign a poor prognosis for anyone with a drug addiction problem, thereby often bypassing addicts in treatment selection.

With the public arousal and concern about drugs, money began to flow into all kinds of drug rehabilitation and prevention programs that were manned by ex-drug addicts who had graduated from Synanon or one of its offshoots such as Daytop or Marathon House. In fact, the professional was excluded in many programs as unable to work effectively with this population. Even if professionals were essential, the problem of numbers of professionals and economics regarding salaries would serve as further barriers. What has gradually occurred now that the emotional upheaval surrounding drug abuse has begun to subside is that the professional is moving in again but this time in a more realistic way as a consultant, trainer-educator, and evaluator-researcher. These roles are more appropriate, using professional manpower to a better degree of efficiency and leaving the day-to-day rehabilitation efforts to lesser trained lay workers with a clinical feel for the problems of the client population that is being served.

Other self-help types of services that fall into this general category are the crisis intervention centers, suicide prevention centers, and drop-in neighborhood clinics. In all of these efforts the manpower problem is solved by using lay persons, volunteers, people living within the target area, and professionals on a consulting, training basis, or as eventual referral sources for the more severely distressed requiring specialized treatment techniques and/or long-term follow-up care. The emphasis is to provide human contact and help on an emergency, easily accessible basis to clients in distress. The traditional nine to five, Monday through Friday mental health facility following extensive intake, diagnostic evaluation, team conference, and treatment plan has fallen short in meeting the needs of people in distress. The community mental health centers have tried to overcome this by extending their services to evening hours and Saturdays. However, like physical illness, crisis of a mental and emotional nature often occurs at inconvenient times such as on weekends, nights, and holidays. The newer crisis-oriented services are providing first aid for mental health problems just as the emergency room of most general hospitals has replaced the private physician in physical crisis situations, especially during the off hours.

Large State-Operated Mental Hospital-Institution Facilities

The large state-operated facility poses many problems that are shared by other similar large public and private institutions. These difficulties can be highlighted more clearly by a discussion of the typical state hospital-type institution. This approach is particularly cogent as there is a developing wave of concern across the country regarding these large facilities. Critics abound in political, professional, and general public domains. The following presentation represents an attempt to analyze some of the factors of growing concern and is a descriptive introductory account of the operation of such institutions.

The prevailing orientation is a defensive one in most state institutions where a closed system exists with efforts directed toward trying to justify programs in the face of glaring unmet needs. Protecting the status quo seems to be the major concern at an administrative as well as political level. "Don't rock the boat" aptly describes, in the vernacular, this type of orientation. The administrator who does not heed this unspoken credo may well find himself/herself under tremendous pressure.

In most of these large state institutions there is an accumulation of inadequate, unmet needs extending over many years. Understaffed, poorly trained, and underpaid personnel operate in overcrowded, inadequate, and frequently physically rundown facilities. Within this system fatalistic attitudes have evolved resulting in treatment that is anti-therapeutic and dehumanizing, reflecting a custodial orientation of aides and other personnel that is subtly passed down from generation to generation. A new worker quickly learns his/her place and any deviation from this prevailing orientation is met with pressures to conform.

On a professional level the quality and numbers of psychiatrists represents a very difficult problem. In the average state hospital most of the medical staff, i.e. physicians, are foreign-born and trained, often in medical schools and at medical centers that do not meet current U. S. medical standards. Training is apt to be heterogeneous among the staff of psychiatrists coming from so many different countries and diverse backgrounds. These doctors are often further handicapped by problems associated with language barriers and cultural differences, factors that are especially important considerations in psychiatry with its emphasis on interpersonal relationships and communication. The selection process is often poor and the quality of psychiatric training and supervision less than optimal in many state institutions. Among many medical and professional groups in the United States, residencies and training programs are assigned low status if they are associated with the state institutional system. As one professional commented to another, who was about to take a job in a state institution, "Why in hell are you going to bury yourself in a state institution?" This clearly reflects a fairly widespread attitude regarding such employment. The result is that the state institution is in a decidedly noncompetitive position in recruitment even when salaries are adequate, which often is not the case. The best psychiatrists following training often leave for more prestigious, lucrative positions especially in private practice.

With respect to some of the other mental health disciplines, the state institution fares a little better, especially if it has university affiliated training programs in such areas as clinical psychology, psychiatric social work, and psychiatric nursing. Quite often the new graduate from these programs can be successfully recruited. However, retaining these professionals becomes a problem as better opportunities quickly open up to them once they complete their graduate training and initiation into the mental health field. Factors that lure such professionals away are better salaries, greater status and prestige within their own professions, and above all, mounting frustrations with the basic job situation. It is extremely difficult not to succumb to inertia, the status quo, and conform to the prevailing orientation of the system, which is decidedly nonprofessional.

For the patient who is committed or must go to a state institution for treatment, he/she has no advocate to insure that his/her rights will not be violated and that adequate, quality treatment will be available. Families of patients still hide in shame, protecting skeletons in the closet regarding a mentally disturbed relative. Even the ex-patient usually wants to hide the history of hospitalization because of job and social discrimination as well as self-devaluation. The general public by and large is apathetic, reacting only when someone raises an emotional outcry that gains media attention. What about the top administrative leaders? The role of advocate conflicts with budgetary limitations, political considerations, and the orientation of defending the status quo. The administrator who speaks out too loudly and too often is very likely to court disfavor from his superiors with a threat of personal chastisement, loss of power, or even dismissal. Advocates for this group will have to come from outside the system or from ex-patients.

The brief historical remarks mentioned at the beginning of this chapter can be reiterated again in this section. The typical state hospital setting is often a dumping grounds for the poor, the disadvantaged, and the unsophisticated. The quality of treatment is poor and the treatment success rate is low. Dependency and institutionalization are still fostered, but to a much lesser degree than in the past, as patients give up the struggle, withdraw, and retreat from the pressures and competition of living in the larger society. The great hope for the breakthrough such as existed when tranquilizers burst on the scene in the early 1950's has never been realized. Patients may adopt the poor prognosis assigned to them in a self-fulfilling prophecy.

For the newly-appointed administrator entering a large state hospital the outlook is indeed very discouraging. He/she will become quickly immersed in a morass of quicksand-type, essentially unsolvable problems. For example, he/she will get caught up with union grievances for better salaries, improved benefits, and working conditions which are beyond the administrator's power to grant. At the same time he/she will be expected to provide some degree of quality service while keeping the costs down. On all levels the new administrator will encounter incompetence, insufficient middle management, and poorly trained line personnel. At best, the new administrator will likely move from one crisis to another and rarely, if ever, have time to really plan or implement a meaningful program. Problems of time, costs, and manpower will obstruct the best of administrators.

What is then the answer to this seemingly impossible situation? In this writer's opinion we are on the threshold of seeing this type of facility phased out. The large, sprawling, self-contained state institution has become archaic. The trend is moving rapidly toward smaller, community-centered facilities, integrated into the community, emphasizing outpatient treatment, brief hospitalization, and keeping the patient near to his/her family and job. The emphasis must be on providing as normal a living situation as possible. In many general hospitals, for example, this has been done for many years quite successfully.

Not only is this trend well established, attempts to revitalize state institutions have repeatedly failed as the system itself contains strong pressures against change, innovation, and efforts to disturb the status quo. Resistance to change is present at all levels, frustrating any efforts to alter the basic anti-therapeutic orientation. Exceptions have been seen mainly in federally sponsored demonstration and/or research projects, newly developed specialized units, and in areas where there is a strong university-state joint affiliation for training professionals such as in social work, clinical psychology, and nursing. New projects and specialized units are usually able to operate somewhat outside the mainstream of the institution, hiring new staff, training them, paying competitive salaries, and creating a more dynamic setting with higher morale and interest in therapeutic procedures.

Thus, it is certainly easier to start by handpicking staff and training them without having to overcome attitudes and behavior patterns that are in conflict with a philosophical outlook of therapeutic treatment. Resistance is not there to thwart and block development and implementation of ideas and procedures. This is in contrast to the rest of the institution where one must work with whomever is already present, regardless of his/her attitudes. The administrator is handicapped by the lack of freedom to fire incompetents, hire new staff, and institute new programs, limitations that often do not exist in a new project or specialized unit.

These projects and specialized units quickly acquire a separate status within the larger institutional structure that results in a lack of integration and minimal impact on changing the overall system. Frequently there is conflict between the two with each viewing the other with distrust or hostility. Once the grant money has ended or the university affiliation has withdrawn, the program and/or unit may be then drawn into the overall institutional structure, but at the same time, lose its vitality and momentum. Key people may leave, of course, with any such changeover, while others may then become frustrated as the entire project is weakened or absorbed into the existing status quo.

Expectations and Pitfalls for the New Administrator

For the newly appointed administrator and student entering the mental health field, words of counsel and advice are perhaps of little value. Direct experience and confrontation with day-to-day happenings within a particular mental health center will do more to shape the views and attitudes of the new administrator or student than any words read in a book, no matter how relevant, incisive, or sage. Notwithstanding this conclusion, some generalized expectations might be of some value, at least as an orientation and preparation for initiation into the mental health field. This preparation may help in avoiding some common problems and point the way for new, more innovative and creative thrusts into this most vital field of human helping.

The novice to mental health settings might first be cautioned to listen to the old-timers, pros, and workers already in the particular setting. Poorly planned changes, even if highly desirable and long overdue, enacted without taking into account the existing structure, methods, and personalities, are bound to be met with much resistance, both open and indirect. Human resistance to change is most important and critical. Failure to recognize this and to appropriately deal with this factor has been the downfall of many administrators, particularly in the mental health field. Passive resistance has plagued many excellently conceived plans. For the new administrator, move slowly at first, making sure you know the organization, its existing structure, its history, and the people who are involved so as to establish creditability and rapport. Try to solicit and encourage their own views on problems and proposals for change and above all, give appropriate recognition of their previous service.

Think through very carefully any changes before implementing them, being attuned to key people in the existing organization and not overlooking anyone who might be slighted or easily threatened. Once again, failure to do so may well be regretted long after the specific change has been implemented or has been superseded by newer policies. Within many organizations, particularly those with political, quasi-political, and public-related affiliation, the power to frustrate and to block programs and progressive changes often rests in the hands of employees at the lowest levels within the organization's heirarchy.

The new administrator should devote an equal amount of time to developing a general philosophy with clearly articulated goals and objectives, well thought out procedures, and policies designed to meet these goals efficiently. Far too many administrators and agencies in the mental health field have no real philosophy. While rules, procedures, and some written objectives are usually available, these are seldom updated, revised, or evaluated in any systematic way until some crisis develops affecting that mental health agency. An organization without meaningful, responsive goals and plans for achieving these goals is apt to be totally unprepared for new ideas and avenues for change from without, reacting only when pressured by forces from without. The locus of change should be from within, but responsive to changes from outside the organization. In essence, stagnatism, lack of innovation, and resistance to responsive change may become the unarticulated orientation.

Armed with (1) viable, realistic, and meaningful goals; (2) a philosophy and a set of action plans for achieving those goals; (3) knowledge of the organization and its staff, and (4) a good rapport with the various personnel, the new administrator is then in a favorable position to initiate change in an orderly, less threatening fashion with greater chances of success. Far too often, the new administrator in his efforts to prove himself moves too quickly, initiates changes without careful preparation, alienates many people, and finds himself caught in a morass of conflict, crisis, and resistance. Once this tragedy has befallen the administrator, it is difficult to correct past errors and regain a position of effective power. Creditability and faith in the administrator's judgment become real issues that affect all of his actions thereafter. Cooperation by subordinates may be impaired, especially critical would be those next in line administratively, who may lose trust in the judgments of the administrator and his programs.

The new administrator, often in his zeal to *administrate*, fails to utilize his subordinates effectively, especially on a supervisory level. Failure to delegate responsibility and to place trust in subordinates inevitably results in a lack of initiative and declining motivation, as well as inefficiency as the administrator becomes increasingly overburdened with trivia and less important duties. Long-range and short-range planning, innovative change, expanding the organization, and improving its functioning may be given less and less serious attention by the administrator under these circumstances. Capable, upwardly mobile supervisory and professional staff are apt to react with frustration and leave the organization for other jobs where their talents and skills will be more appreciated and better utilized.

Along with the delegation of authority and responsibility there should be a careful, tactful approach to following up on these delegated duties, amply rewarding accomplishments, and guiding further similar efforts. Follow through is as essential as delegation to insure that the assignments have been fulfilled within a reasonable period of time with a maximum of efficiency. Accountability must always be a necessary handmaiden to the delegation of responsibility and authority. Without some external structuring, unpleasant, difficult tasks have a way of becoming bogged down, procrastinated upon, sidelined, and otherwise not completed or avoided completely. There may also be a tendency for the subordinate to lose sight of the original areas of responsibility, resulting in unplanned conflicts and problems. In short, an effective administrator does not hesitate to delegate responsibility and to give that person ample freedom to fulfill that charge by offering guidance, support, and structure so that there is an accountability, follow-up, and appropriate evaluation.

Working with professionals poses some unique problems for the administrator in the mental health field. Most professionals demand and expect a considerable amount of personal freedom in fulfilling their jobs. Independence, especially along professional lines, is extremely important for the self-esteem of most professionals. In general, professionals do not like to be told how to do their work, conform to many rules and regulations, or feel that their input into the organization is unimportant, taken for granted, or ignored. Professional freedom is absolutely essential with opportunities to grow, develop new ideas, and engage in creative work. The administrator, whether he/she be a professional administrator or mental health professional, who fails to appreciate this basic factor is bound to encounter difficulties in dealing with professional workers. This is not to say that the administrator has to coddle or make undue allowances for *temperamental, creative* professionals, but he/she must be prepared to appreciate the importance of personal freedom to most professionals, approaching them on an equal, mature level, and avoid talking down to them.

Notwithstanding the foregoing commentary about the professional, of course, there should be limits placed on activities, basic rules to follow, and accountability with consequences for overstepping certain privileges, which apply equally to the professional, and to anyone else within the organization. The point being emphasized is the method of approach and the attitude of the administrator toward the professional worker. A mistake of many administrators in all types of administrative settings is the error of treating everyone alike or assuming that everyone should be or is like the administrator himself. Individual differences are a fact of life and the administrator whose primary function is administrating people must not ignore this without paying distressing consequences.

An effective administrator must also create an atmosphere of security and stability while keeping the organization open to innovation and change. He/she must lead, guide, direct, and create an atmosphere in which change is expected, encouraged, and not resisted. Any organization that becomes closed eventually stagnates, loses its vitality, and invites pressures from outside the system for change. Its goals become hazy, its mission unclear, and it becomes unresponsive to ongoing change.

A last point of advice to the new administrator concerns the hiring of staff, promotions, and assignments. Caution is the key. Be sure you know your candidates well; do not hire or promote anyone because it is expedient at the moment. An incompetent worker, supervisor, or person who differs widely from the general goals of the organization may become the source of many problems in the future. How often have we seen a person hired because of a critical shortage who later thwarts and impedes the progress of the organization because of incompetence, differing philosophy, and/or personality problems. Meeting an immediate need may be greatly overshadowed in the long run if the administrator has hired or promoted the wrong person. It is easier not to hire or not to promote someone than it is to later fire or demote that person, which frequently occurs only after much invested time, difficult personal confrontations, aroused emotions, and damaged morale.

Frequently the administrator finds himself stuck with a resistant employee whom he cannot dismiss without undue friction. There is no easy solution to this problem, although it is recommended that first efforts be made to work with the employee, win his confidence, and bring him into the mainstream of the organization. If failure to succeed along these lines occurs, then the administrator might try to bypass and/or neutralize this person's resistance by concentrating efforts on the remaining surrounding staff. The final step may involve direct confrontation in the form of a notice to the employee to make specific changes, and ultimately, to suspension or dismissal. Sometimes before this last stage is reached, the person will cooperate sufficiently, withdraw voluntarily, leave to retire, move onto another job, or terminate due to illness. Once any key position is vacated, careful screening in replacing this position cannot be overemphasized. This is especially important in filling supervisory and professional positions.

Conclusions

In this chapter we have tried to focus upon the problems that the newly-appointed administrator and student might anticipate in the mental health field. To conclude this presentation with a practical orientation, some of the key areas that need redress can be summarized. Scanning the field of mental health services one sees (1) an excessive duplication of services, (2) inadequate interagency communication and coordination, (3) outdated models for delivery of services, (4) a lack of innovativeness and creativity in agency goals and organization, (5) underutilization of lesser trained staff in treatment, (6) a need for better trained administrators, (7) little use of modern business cost-efficiency techniques, and (8) few advocates for the client population of emotionally disturbed.

From this list there is much that can be and needs to be done in the field of mental health, especially from an administrator's perspective. For example, demonstration-type projects need to become more than subsidized grants, essentially duplicating existing services. More innovation and creativity are needed as existing models are failing to provide a quality of services that really meet clients' needs in an expanding population. Even with regard to basic research, more socially relevant studies directed toward mental health problems of real people is needed to supplement the more tightly controlled, laboratory research study. Relevance to current social problems is central to this recommendation. Service agencies should try to draw upon social science researchers as consultants or even full-salaried employees. Such a blend would give a more balanced perspective, resulting in greater innovativeness, a reapproachment between the researcher and clinician to the growth of both, and ultimately, to the benefit of the patient in distress through improvement in the quality of services.

REFERENCES

Bockoven, J. S.: Moral treatment in American psychiatry. *J Nerv Ment Dis,* 124:167-194, 292-321, 1956.

Bruch, H.: *Eating Disorders: Obesity, Anorexia Nervosa and the Person Within.* New York, Basic Books, 1973.

Coleman, J. C. and Broen, W. E. Jr.: *Abnormal Psychology and Modern Life.* Glenview, 1972.

Diagnostic and Statistical Manual of Mental Disorders. Washington, D. C., American Psychiatric Association, 1968.

Goldenberg, H.: *Contemporary Clinical Psychology.* Monterey, Brooks/ Cole Publishing, 1973.

Heckman, I. L. Jr., and Huneryager, S. G.: *Human Relations in Management.* Cincinnati, South-Western Publishing, 1960.

Joint Commission on Mental Illness and Health: *Action for Mental Health.* New York, Basic Books, 1961.

Mayer, J.: *Overweight: Causes, Cost, and Control.* Englewood Cliffs, Prentice-Hall, 1968.

Shakow, D.: *Clinical Psychology as Science and Profession: A Forty-Year Odyssey.* Chicago, Aldine Publishing, 1969.

Taulbee, E. S. and Wright, H. W.: A psychosocial-behavioral model for therapeutic intervention. In Spielberger, C. D. (Ed.): *Current Topics in Clinical and Community Psychology.* New York, Academic Press, 1971.

Chapter 3

SERVING THE MENTALLY RETARDED IN REHABILITATION FACILITIES

Leon Meenach

Meeting the Facility Needs of the Mentally Retarded in Rehabilitation Facilities

REHABILITATION FACILITIES represent a valuable resource in modern day rehabilitation practice. Facilities provide the means for evaluating, treating and training the severely disabled who otherwise could not be effectively rehabilitated. In this case, we are referring to the mentally retarded whose employment opportunities can be enhanced by participating in facility services.

Facilities come in all sizes and scope of program. All disability groups may be served in a single facility or only selected groups. We will devote this chapter to facilities services designed for or available to the mentally retarded. Usually you find two types of facilities—medically oriented and vocationally oriented. We will be concerned primarily with the vocationally oriented facility services for the mentally retarded. The modern rehabilitation facility today will have available a full range of services that can be brought to bear on the needs of the client.

Various approaches have been made in the past years toward integration of the mentally retarded into the mainstream of productivity with varying degrees of success. Many meritorious efforts to habilitate or rehabilitate this large disability group have been limited. The comprehensive facility and the community workshop have provided us with one of the most valuable tools to effectively meet the needs of this group. Before going further, we should explore who the mentally retarded are.

Who Are the Retarded?

The mentally retarded are children and adults who, as a result of inadequately developed intelligence, are significantly impaired in ability to learn and to adapt to the demands of society. The mentally retarded youth often experience great difficulty in making the transition from school to work. School dropout rates and other indicators of personal disorganization, such as rates of delinquency, are high. Oftentimes rejected by family and society, faced with a future of failure, defeated before they have the opportunity to begin, these young people feel like social discards.

The retarded are targets of degrading experience, their judgment is poor, they are submissive and on the receiving end of cruel jokes and many times the scapegoat in criminal activities. The retarded are also persons with much the same feelings, aspirations, problems, desires and characteristics as any other member of society.

Most definitions for mental retardation refer to intellectual function, adaptive behavior, and deviation from the norm. The most generally quoted definition is that developed by the American Association of Mental Deficiency and is quoted as follows: "Mental retardation refers to significantly sub-average intellectual functioning which manifests itself during the developmental period and is characterized by inadequacy and/or inadaptive behavior."

Eligibility for Services

Most facilities that provide services for the mentally retarded are either referred by state agency counselors or the referral originates at the facility workshop and then is brought to the attention of the VR counselor for consideration of eligibility and feasibility for VR sponsorship. A number of facilities may serve a combination of mentally retarded clients who are sponsored by VR state agencies as well as those mentally retarded who do not have potential for gainful employment.

Vocational rehabilitation state agencies use IQ and functional factors in determining which clients can be served and deciding on an individual basis. The disability may manifest itself as subnormality in the following areas:

A. Intellectual functioning
B. Academic achievement

C. Rate of learning

D. Social or emotional maturity

E. Adaptability in job preparation

The VR counselor establishes eligibility on the basis of psychological, vocational and social evaluations. The vocational evaluation aspect is usually documented in the case history in some detail considering previously adjudged mentally retarded, personal inadequacies, educational inadequacies, and vocational inadequacies.

Possible client categories according to vocational potential and capacity for self-care are:

A. Capable of competitive employment and independent living

B. Capable of competitive employment but needs supervised living arrangements

C. Needs sheltered employment and needs supervised living arrangements

D. No vocational potential but capable of supervised living

E. Institutional care

Vocational rehabilitation will more than likely be active in the habilitation and rehabilitation needs of the first three groups.

Generally speaking, vocational rehabilitation works effectively with all who have vocational potential as shown by pre-vocational and vocational evaluation coupled with proper training. Experience seems to indicate 50-55 to be the possible lower score while 80-85 tends to find less services as a group.

Vocational Implications of Serving the Mentally Retarded

Experience leads us to believe that actual or specific vocational choice is of little importance as long as we can lead the client to accept realistic areas of work. Factors of great importance are motivation, personality, work attitudes and traits, use of leisure time and social maturity. There are a lot of factors or implications to consider and cope with during the rehabilitation process. There may be associated mental problems, such as epilepsy or others. The availability of work has serious implications in job development. The mentally retarded tend to be "last hired and first fired or laid off if there is an economic slump." We tend to select the menial routine type jobs for this group. The greatest success has been in low paying jobs, e.g. janitor, mail clerk, busboy, messenger, laundry worker. But these aren't the only type jobs available to the mentally retarded. He may have a slow rate of learning but many can achieve normal levels of vocational attainment; it just simply takes longer. Menial tasks can also be performed with dignity and pride.

Professionals, employers, and friends dealing with the mentally retarded will have to possess a large measure of patience, understanding and foresight. Some of the higher level mentally retarded are able to feel, and to a degree, recognize their limitations while at the same time they have feelings and aspirations much the same as their normal neighbors.

Facility Programs for the Retarded

Facility services developed or anticipated should account for the clients' individual needs in light of his assets and liabilities and provide him with whatever vocationally relevant services are needed to help him become employed. Business and industry seek persons who can meet particular characteristics of a job. The facility can serve this group who are mentally retarded and have difficulties in making adjustment. The facility or workshop programming must be geared to a level of their understanding and abilities. Their frustration tolerances are sometimes lower and behavioral problems are present. Tasks presented must be in small enough increments to be handled and must be repeated many times.

Any facility dealing with the retarded must be flexible enough to allow for individual differences and for recycling if needed by a client who misses an important step which will be a problem to him at some time in the future.

Most rehabilitation workshops are transitional and serve all groups of the disabled. You will find a large percentage of the mentally retarded are in workshops or work activity centers. A smaller number are usually found in the large comprehensive centers. There is also the need for workshop activity and extended employment for those mentally retarded not readily acceptable to the employment market but productive at below level of performance.

Facilities and workshops serving the mentally retarded have been innovative in their ability to provide services. Behavior modification techniques have been very productive where behavior becomes a problem as well as absenteeism and task completion.

There isn't basically a difference in types of evaluation for the mentally retarded client. We must take into account the individual differences and the level of function and other factors pertinent to finding out what an individual's assets and liabilities are. We need to determine how to build on assets and/or overcome the liabilities. Different approaches and tools however may be necessary.

Facility Administration When Serving the Retarded

It is important for the facility that provides services for the retarded to build a two-way communication system between the client sponsor and the facility. Communication and feedback between the sponsor (rehabilitation counselor) and the facility staff is the most important responsibility in achieving the goal of providing the best services for the mentally retarded client. The vocational rehabilitation state agency staff, which includes the counselor, should continually discuss policies regarding the scope of services offered, legal limitations and obligations, as well as various fee schedules or contract arrangements that exist between the two staffs. All parties should insure that the client is receiving full benefits of effective and responsive services. The two-way communication should be an objective and a frank basis which allows for open discussion with mutual trust.

The Georgia rehabilitation agency approaches this need for involvement through the use of a planning cycle approach. The community facilities and the VR agency recognizes the desirability of encouraging stable, meaningful programs in rehabilitation facilities operated by private, nonprofit groups. In order to foster their stability and provide increasingly better services to the disabled client, the agency and facility enters into an agreement mutually beneficial to the client, facility and VR agency.

A joint planning meeting is held prior to the initiation or revision of agreements or charges involving appropriate members of the facility staff and local VR agency staff. To insure that the services are needed, responsive, and can be fully utilized, the following considerations are taken into account at the planning meetings in April and May of each year:

1. Program design of the rehabilitation facility and services which can be provided to clients sponsored.
2. Client capacity of the facility.
3. Number of clients anticipated by the agency in the geographical location served by the facility.
4. Cost of operating the rehabilitation facility (or that part of the facility serving VR clients or a special disability group).

The agreements are reduced to budget form with agreement in principle by both the VR agency and the facility of the quality and quantity of services which can be furnished. Constant review and evaluation of the programs are carried out jointly for the purpose of considering modifications which are desirable to both parties.

Approaches similar to this can be helpful to the administrators in planning, programming and budget for a productive program of services that will be utilized for the mentally retarded client.

The facility administrator must be aware of both positive and negative attitudes of clients, staff, self, employers, and counselors. Staff should be selected carefully and approach the clients and others with tender, sensitive, direct and persuasive counsel as the case calls for. This approach is an essential ingredient in serving the retarded.

There will be a need for staff to have some skills to deal with special individuals of behavior deviating from the norm and other areas of adjustment. All staff must make allies of the mentally retarded client by persuasive counsel and solicitation of their energies toward positive goals rather than contributing to the problem.

The administrator and his staff, in order to effectively serve the mentally retarded in a facility need to be patient and flexible and have endurance and understanding plus the ability to communicate at all levels and be able to feel for the "unloved" and "unlovable."

Conclusion

Serving the mentally retarded in rehabilitation facilities is basically similar to most facilities where assessment and diagnosis take place. The client is exposed to a general evaluation where work samples, situational assessment, testing, work activity, personal adjustment, and training are provided. What may be expected, special is the provision of relevant, realistic and helpful services which are based on individual needs, aspirations, desires and which assists the mentally retarded client toward a reachable and profitable goal. That he can achieve a measure of success while living through the experiences of his present environment (the facility) and that he can be reasonably happy while seeking achievement. That he is trained, urged, pointed toward, or otherwise moved in the direction of something (job) that is available when he completes his facility program. That we discharge him in a better condition than we found him.

CHAPTER 4

PROVIDING SERVICES TO ALCOHOLICS THROUGH REHABILITATION FACILITIES

A. HOWARD BELL

IT HAS NOT BEEN too long ago that the rehabilitation of alcoholics merely involved drying them out in a drunk tank in jail or detoxifying them in a hospital, if they could get in, then sending them back home and to work.* Those who were afflicted might have tried to alter their drinking behavior in certain ways, such as limiting the amount of alcohol consumption or by staying away from the *hard stuff* (e.g. bourbon and scotch) only to end up in repeated failure and frustration. He or she was thought to be either a skid row bum or delinquent or seen as a weak-willed individual who couldn't hold his liquor like a man or drink like a lady, whichever the case may be. This was the general view of the alcoholic that was held prior to 1940, and is still held today to a larger extent than we like to admit.

During the Alumni Institute of the Summer School of Alcohol Studies at Rutgers University, Dr. Seldon Bacon (1972) pointed out in a talk to the participants that prior to 1940, we had the protagonists. For example, he noted there were the "wets vs. the drys" and there were pro and con arguments about the nature of alcohol and its effects on the body. He added there were some exceptions, however, such as the attitude taken by the Salvation Army and a scattering of physicians and hospitals. Then between 1940 and 1945, when the Center of Alcoholic Studies was established, there emerged a scientific approach. He said that the goal of this approach was to "cast off the shackles" of the past and to initiate a systematic and organized attack on

---

* A notable exception to this statement has been the activities on a nonprofessional level of Alcoholics Anonymous since its founding in 1935, by Bill W. and Dr. Bob S.

the nature of alcoholism. Although the "new look" that *alcoholism is a disease* was being circulated at that time, about fifteen years was to pass before E. M. Jellinek (1960) published his book entitled *The Disease Concept of Alcoholism*.

Comparing the early 1940's with the early 1970's, Bacon (1972) noted that in 1941 and 1942, there were hardly enough articles to publish in the *Quarterly Journal of Studies on Alcohol*. In 1970, this journal was publishing ten issues a year instead of the usual four, and the present writer can vouch that in 1970 there was a one-year waiting period between the submission of an article and its publication date. Bacon also called attention to the fact that in 1940, there was next to nothing about alcoholism in the news media except that which was negative. At the various kinds of professional meetings, alcoholism was generally ridiculed, as if the term *alcoholic* were a dirty word. Currently, however, the situation has changed considerably. The United States Congress and the legislatures in every state in the Union are spending money to set up programs for diagnosis, treatment, training, and research in the field of alcoholism. Professional organizations, such as the American Psychological Association, are holding symposia on alcoholism, and all the mass news media are cooperating in an effort to deal constructively with this problem.

Thus during the past thirty to thirty-five years, the portrayal of the alcoholic has undergone a slow but definite change from the typical derelict or *weak sister* image to the view that alcoholics are sick people. Along with this conceptual change, there has been a positive shift in attitude on the American scene as regards treatment and rehabilitation opportunities for the alcoholic. Spearheading this change, of course, was the Yale University Center of Alcohol Studies in New Haven, Connecticut and more recently the Rutgers University Center of Alcohol Studies, with its Summer School of Alcohol Studies, in New Brunswick, New Jersey. Also, the position taken by the World Health Organization (WHO) and the American Medical Association (AMA) that alcoholism is an illness has given substantial (and some would say even *critical*) support to both the medical and the social nature of this condition. For example, WHO (Schmidt,

1952) has taken the stance that "alcoholics are those excessive drinkers whose dependence upon alcohol has attained such a degree that it shows a noticeable mental disturbance or an interference with their bodily and mental health, their interpersonal relations, and their smooth social and economic functioning; or who show prodromal signs of such development. They therefore require treatment."

As one might suspect from the above description of the alcoholic, most of the alcoholics in the United States who fit this definition would more frequently be our neighbors next door than the chronic homeless drunk on the street. Indeed, it has been estimated that only about 3 to 5 percent of the alcoholic population are denizens of the skid-rows across the country (Eaton, 1972).

Demographic Characteristics and Personality Patterns

Demographic Characteristics

Since alcoholism affects women as well as men, in both rural and urban areas and without regard for cultural background, religious preference, educational level, or financial standing, it is easy to see how the majority of this country's alcoholics could be one's friends and acquaintances, one's next-door neighbor, so to speak. A study (Bell *et al.*, 1969) which involved a sampling of thirty-seven white male alcoholics who were participating in the alcoholism program at East Louisiana State Hospital in Jackson clearly supports the observation that neither intellectual level nor socioeconomic status, whether high, medium, or low, is a barrier to the development of the illness called alcoholism. The demographic and levels of intelligence data are noted in the following paragraph.

Regarding intellectual level, it was found that IQ scores obtained from the Shipley-Hartford Vocabulary Test, ranged from a low of 79, and extended up to and including a high of 140. The average IQ score of this distribution was 102. The age range of this sample of patients was twenty-seven years to sixty-three years inclusive. In spite of the apparent favorable age factor for marriage, only 38 percent were married. Forty-three percent of this group were either separated or divorced, and 8 percent were widowers. Eleven percent were single and had never been married. Regarding occupational level, it was found that 22 percent of these subjects were either professional men or business executives, for example, an engineer or contractor. Fifty-seven percent were skilled workers, such as bricklayers or carpenters. Sixteen percent were semiskilled workers, for example, service station attendant, and only 5 percent were unskilled laborers. Additional data showed that 92 percent of these patients had been arrested at least once in their lives for operating a motor vehicle while under the influence of alcohol or for simple drunkenness. Of this group of patients, 70 percent were voluntary admissions, and the remaining 30 percent were committed by the coroner* in response to a request that was usually made by the family of the alcoholic. As for prior hospitalizations, 68 percent had been hospitalized for alcoholism before, either at East Louisiana State Hospital or someplace else. Concerning Alcoholics Anonymous, approximately 43 percent had previous exposure (one or more meetings) to the AA program.

The picture shifts somewhat when these kinds of data are looked at in relation to the number of previous admissions to an alcoholism treatment program. That is, when one compares data obtained on first-admission alcoholics with data obtained from the recidivist (four or more admissions), notable, and in some cases, dramatic, changes are observed in such categories as average age, marital status, occupational level, residence factors, frequency of blackouts and/or delirium tremens and post-hospitalization plans. The following discussion of these changes is based upon a partial extraction of data obtained on a group of white male alcoholics which are contained in an unpublished study (Bell and Weingold, 1968) also conducted at East Louisiana State Hospital. This study revealed that the average age of first-admission patients was forty-three years as compared with the recidivist of fifty years. Fifty-five percent of the first-admission alcoholics were married, 34 percent were separated or divorced,

---

* In Louisiana commitment proceedings are processed by the Coroner of a given parish (county).

4 percent were widowed, and 7 percent single. Fifty-nine percent of the repeaters were married, and 41 percent were either separated or divorced; there were no widowers nor single subjects in this group. The level of occupation shifts only slightly from 54 percent for the skilled workers (including professional and business people) and 46 percent for the non-skilled to 47 percent and 53 percent, respectively. As concerns residence factors, in the first-admission group, 59 percent lived with their wives, 30 percent lived with a relative or friend, and the remaining 11 percent lived by themselves (alone). With the "swinging door" group, 67 percent lived with their wives, only 13 percent lived with relatives or friends, but 20 percent lived alone. As regards blackouts and D.T.'s, quite noticeable changes take place among the first-admission alcoholics; 37 percent had experienced blackouts but not D.T.'s; only 7 percent had experienced D.T.'s but not blackouts; 14 percent had experienced both, but the largest group, *42 percent, had experienced neither blackouts nor D.T.'s*. In contrast, just 18 percent of the recidivists had experienced blackouts but not D.T.'s; 23 percent had experienced D.T.'s but not blackouts; however, the majority of patients, 59 percent, had experienced *both* blackouts *and* D.T.'s. Thus, it can be seen that 100 percent of those patients who were admitted four or more times for treatment *had experienced either blackouts or D.T.'s or both*. Finally, regarding motivation, as might be reflected in the patients' post-hospitalization plans to attend meetings of Alcoholics Anonymous, 57 percent of the first-admission group planned to continue to go to AA meetings following discharge; the remaining 43 percent had no AA plans. However, there was a noticeable difference in the percentage of patients in the recidivists' group who planned to go to AA, as compared to those who had no AA plans. Specifically, 71 percent had AA plans, and only 29 percent did not. These data are summarized in Table I.

Personality Patterns

Since it has been observed that alcoholics as a group display certain distinctive behavioral patterns, the question arises, "Is there an 'alcoholic personality'?" Some of the personality traits

TABLE I

A COMPARISON OF RECIDIVIST VS. FIRST-ADMISSION ALCOHOLICS
ON AVERAGE AGE, MARITAL STATUS, OCCUPATIONAL LEVEL,
RESIDENCE FACTORS, FREQUENCY OF BLACKOUTS AND/OR
D.T.'S, AND POST-HOSPITALIZATION PLANS*

First Admission *Mean Age* (N=47) .... 43 yrs. *Percentage*		*Four or More Admissions* *Mean Age* (N=17) .... 50 yrs. *Percentage*	
Marital Status (N=47)		*Marital Status* (N=17)	
Married	55	Married	59
Separated or Divorced	34	Separated or Divorced	41
Widowed	4	Widowed	0
Single	7	Single	0
Occupational Level (N=46)		*Occupational Level* (N=17)	
Skilled	54	Skilled	47
Non-Skilled	46	Non-Skilled	53
Residence Factors (N=44)		*Residence Factors* (N=15)	
Lives With Wife	59	Lives With Wife	67
Lives With Relative or Friend	30	Lives With Relative or Friend	13
Lives Alone	11	Lives Alone	20
Blackouts and D.T.'s (N=43)		*Blackouts and D.T.'s* (N=17)	
Blackouts Only	37	Blackouts Only	18
D.T.'s Only	7	D.T.'s Only	23
Both Blackouts and D.T.'s ..	14	Both Blackouts and D.T.'s ..	59
Neither Blackouts nor D.T.'s	42	Neither Blackouts nor D.T.'s	0
Post-Hospitalization Plans (N=46)		*Post-Hospitalization Plans* (N=17)	
AA Plans	57	AA Plans	71
No AA Plans	43	No AA Plans	29

* Data obtained from an unpublished study conducted by A. Howard Bell and Harold P. Weingold, 1968.

suggested by the behavior of the alcoholic are impulsiveness, resentfulness, hypersensitivity to criticism, lack of self-confidence, rebelliousness, aggressiveness, suspiciousness, passivity, feelings of guilt, and the persistent use of the defense mechanisms of rationalization (alibis) and denial. An element of depression is also found in a large percentage of alcoholics. For example, Weingold et al. (1968) studied seventy-three consecutively admitted alcoholics to an alcoholism treatment program of a large state hospital and found that 70 percent of the subjects exhibited mild to deep depression.

However, there are a lot of other people with these same characteristics who never become alcoholics. Therefore, such personality traits could hardly be the exclusive property of the alcoholic implied in "the alcoholic personality" label. Yet clusters of various combinations of personality traits keep popping-up in the alcoholic population, which suggest that practicing alcoholics (i.e. those alcoholics who are still drinking or who have been "dry" for a relatively short period of time) as a group at least, have certain common behavioral traits; whereas a particular personality trait or combination of personality traits may be pronounced in a given alcoholic, in another they might not be.

Indeed, in an investigation conducted by Lawlis and Rubin (1971), three different groups of alcoholics were identified. In this study, the intercorrelations of the personality profiles, obtained from the Sixteen Personality Factor (16-PF) Questionnaire, were factor analyzed. All three groups were found to be emotionally unstable, but there were certain significant group characteristics that distinguished each group from the others. For example, the group that was classified as *inhibited* was apprehensive, tense, and shy. The group that was labeled as *sociopathic* was shrewd, conservative, and evaded rules; and the group that was described as *aggressive* had high scores on aggression, tough-mindedness, and suspiciousness. Thus, as the investigators concluded, these results appear to cast serious doubt about the concept of *the* alcoholic personality.

Taken one step further, since the concept of personality is viewed as unique to the individual and since it is likely that separate personality types would emerge using a different (from the 16-PF) personality test, an argument might even be made that there are as many alcoholic personalities as there are alcoholics. Hence, it is felt that the most we can say, at this stage of the game, is that there is a maladaptive adjustment factor common to all alcoholics, which is exactly what we presumed in the first place.

Working With the Alcoholic: Some Problems Encountered

It appears to me that the most difficult problem that a person (a helper) who is working with an alcoholic (a helpee) is faced with centers around the mechanisms of rationalization and denial—defenses that the alcoholic has become an expert at using. With reference to the alcoholic, the term "rationalization" simply means finding reasons (alibis, excuses) that are acceptable to himself, and hopefully to others, for his drinking behavior. For example, on a given occasion he may say he got drunk because he was celebrating his promotion or because he got fired and was drowning his sorrows. He may think himself into believing that he drinks because the children make him nervous, or in his later years because he is very lonely since the children grew up, got married, and moved away. He may rationalize that he is a veteran who served his country in time of war and now has a service-connected disability and deserves to get soused to the gill. He may think that he has the right to drink because the wife nags him all the time. In the case of a female alcoholic, she may say she drinks because her husband takes her for granted and because he values his job more than he does her and the family. The alcoholic may argue that he has to drink in order to overcome certain social inferiorities that he believes he has, or that he drinks in order to make the right kind of connections in business. He might be heard to say, "What's the matter with drinking? Everybody does it!" To be sure, if the alcoholic has decided that he is going to drink, he will find a reason.

Sooner or later, the alcoholic may be hard pressed to alibi his way out of a particular situation. Yet it may be that the alcoholic's *alibi system* might never collapse; i.e. he may never completely run out of excuses for drinking. If so, so much the worse for him. On the other hand, his alibi system could collapse, but if new and constructive behavioral changes do not take the place of the old destructive drinking behavior, the system is likely to be rebuilt. In other words, when the collapse occurs and alibis fail to do the job of preventing the alcoholic from accepting the reality that he has a problem associated with alcohol, the alcoholic is most accessible and amenable to treatment. AA members oftentimes refer to this stage of the alcoholic's drinking career as "hitting bottom." At an AA convention one time, an AA member told the story about the last time he was hospitalized for alcoholism. After he was admitted, he was given a hospital gown to put on that exposed very nearly his entire backside. He walked down the hall to look at himself in a full length mirror, and when he turned around in front of the mirror to check the loosely tied strings on the back of his gown, he exclaimed that he had not only reached his bottom, he saw it!

Strange as it may seem, however, hospitalization or a commitment doesn't necessarily bring about a collapse of the alibi system. In the late 1960's, when I was employed as the Chief Psychologist of a large mental hospital, one of my assignments was to conduct all of the intake staff conferences on the alcoholism treatment service. Since one of the primary goals of the alcoholism program was to help the patient to accept the reality of his situation, I would ask each of them if he or she thought that he or she were an alcoholic. If the reply happened to be negative, I would ask them, "What is an alcoholic, anyway?" Should the answer be something like, "Well, I don't know exactly," I would reply with something similar to, "If you don't really know what an alcoholic is, then how do you know you're not one?" If they still denied they were alcoholic, I would ask them if they thought they might have a *drinking problem*. Should the answer again be "no," I would ask them, "If you don't believe you are an alcoholic nor that you have a drinking problem, would you, at least, admit that drinking has caused you some problems?" Surprisingly enough, in spite of the fact that the interviewees were patients in a mental institution, albeit an alcoholism ward, at times I would also get a "no" response to this last question. Finally, when I would ask the patient, "You say you are not an alcoholic, you don't have a drinking problem, and drinking has not caused you any problems, yet you are a patient in a state hospital due to your drinking behavior, and that's no problem?" In this case, sometimes (but not always) a patient might reluctantly admit his current situation presents certain problems.

Thus we can easily see that the defense of denial is closely associated with the mechanism of rationalization. When an alcoholic rationalizes, when he gives what may seem to him to be a plausible reason for his drinking, he is indirectly denying that he has a drinking problem. Direct denial is manifested when the alcoholic refuses to admit, even to himself, that he has a drinking problem. In spite of the obvious (to others) signs of a problem, such as arrests for driving while under the influence of alcohol (or other mood altering drugs), arrests for simple drunkenness, separation or divorce stemming from drinking behavior, loss of friends, loss of occupational or professional licenses, the loss of a good credit rating, and blackouts, despite these glaring signals, the alcoholic may still be unable to recognize the seriousness of his problem and/or be unwilling to admit that he is "one of those" alcoholics.

Physical Disability vs. Alcoholic Disability

Some Theoretical Considerations

Contrary to the point of view that is generally held by rehabilitation counselors and other rehabilitation workers, it has been theorized elsewhere (Bell, 1970) that whether the mechanism of denial results in positive or negative consequences depends upon the type of disability with which we are dealing and the psychological adjustment stage that the afflicted individual has reached in the rehabilitation process. In other words, where physical disability is concerned, as opposed to alcoholic disability, in the initial phase of rehabilitation, denial could have positive consequences from a long-range point of view. The phases I am referring to are the stages I have observed in the adjustment of the chronically ill or disabled person. The first stage oftentimes involves denial or non-acceptance of the condition. Closely associated with denial there may be a second stage of frustration, manifested by either hostile and aggressive behavior or depression (which is considered to be merely aggressive tendencies turned inward toward the self). Following denial and frustration, a third stage of intellectual recognition and admission of the problem may present itself. Then lastly, the fourth stage of emotional acceptance, hopefully, appears. It has been my experience that a client may progress through each one of these stages as outlined, or he may get stuck at, say, the first and second stages and never reach the stage of emotional acceptance.

Or he may reach the point of acceptance, but in an emotional crisis he may revert back to an earlier stage.

Let me give you an example of a client in the first and second stages of adjustment. Several years ago I was acquainted with a beautiful twenty-one-year-old young lady in the prime of her life who became paralyzed in both lower extremities as the result of an unfortunate automobile accident. Following hospitalization, she was sent to a rehabilitation center for a program of physical therapy. After a few months of treatment she was told by the physiatrist that she would never walk again. Since the patient was adjusting to her condition with denial (non-acceptance), this disclosure by her doctor engendered within the patient a great deal of anger and hostility. She just could not believe that she would never walk again. The result was that she tried all the more to prove that she (the patient) was right and would walk again and that the doctor was wrong. Therefore, it is speculated that the effect of denial that the patient was displaying acted as a motivational factor that energized a strong desire to improve. Shortly afterwards, the patient was discharged from the rehabilitation center with "maximum therapeutic benefits." However, she continued her physical therapy regime at home, and a year or so later this girl took a taxi downtown and went shopping unassisted by friends or relatives. After three long arduous years, she walked. With the aid of crutches and braces, it's true, but she walked!

In the foregoing case it is felt that without the defense of denial as a motivating factor, there might be some question as to whether this patient would have attained the amount of return that she experienced or the level of physical restoration and rehabilitation that she achieved. Eventually, when denial had spent its usefulness, of course, the patient needed to shift her denial to an attitude of acceptance in order to attain an optimal level of adjustment. However, in the beginning stages of her recovery and rehabilitation, it is proposed that denial had served a useful purpose.

Such is not the case where alcoholism is concerned. Bell

(1970) noted that it is conceivable that denial of the problem could prevent the alcoholic from ever recovering from his condition. As long as the denial persists, and the alcoholic does not desire to stop drinking, chances are he will continue to drink. Thus it would seem that the first order of business with the counselor who is working with an alcoholic would be to assist the alcoholic in his struggle to determine the existence of the problem by using so-called "directive" techniques along with empathy and understanding. The family could assist by using the doctrine of *tough love* in their relationship with the alcoholic. Tough love involves a display of love for the afflicted party but with a stance of nonacceptance of his drinking (alcoholic) behavior, including his alibies. If the alcoholic is unwilling to seek the help that he needs in spite of a tough love policy, a crisis may need to be created by manipulating the environment in order to get the patient into an institution for proper treatment. If necessary, commitment is one alternative. Thus, if the alcoholic hasn't reached his bottom, as the AA's put it, then there are ways of raising his bottom so that he can reach it.

Following the admission of the problem and as the recovery process progresses, the alcoholic should "begin to accept his condition realistically, not only in terms of its conscious recognition, but also in terms of an accepting attitude toward the self and the condition, which would be reflected in his living successfully as a rehabilitated alcoholic" (Bell *et al.*, 1969). A scale, "The Bell Alcoholism Scale of Adjustment," designed to measure the extent of acceptance has been described elsewhere (Bell *et al.*, 1969; Bell, 1970).

The point that I am trying to make here is that although the generality of the significance of the role of acceptance applies to both physical disability and to alcoholism (or to all chronic disabling conditions, for that matter), acceptance of a disability may not necessarily be reflected in a totally positive behavioral pattern (Bell, 1967; Bell, 1970). That is to say, a person with a disabling condition who is adjusting to that condition as a passive acceptor, as distinct from an active acceptor, will not be motivated to help himself. With physical disability, the passive acceptor would be too dependent and would let others do things for him that he could do for himself. With alcoholism, the passive acceptor responds as if to say, "Okay, I'm an alcoholic, so I can't control my drinking," then proceeds to go out and get drunk. The active acceptor, on the other hand, does something positive about his condition. The physically disabled active acceptor would accept his identity with the disabled population but would try to be as independent as possible and to live as normal a life as his limitations would permit. The alcoholic, who is an active acceptor, would accept his condition and would be motivated to seek a satisfying way of life *sans* alcohol, i.e. as an abstinent (sober) alcoholic.

Hence, from the viewpoint of long-range goals, acceptance of one's disability would not be the only, nor invariably the most desirable, attitude the counselor would want to instill in a client (Bell and Stickel, 1971). The key, of course, is the factor of motivation, which may come spontaneously in the guise of denial for the physically disabled person. The moral here is for counselors who are working with the physically disabled to stop saying "If he would only accept his condition, he would be all right and be a good patient," and start using the patient's denial as a motivating force. For the alcoholic, though, denial merely delays the achievement of the maximum benefits from the overall rehabilitation effort. If contented sobriety is the goal, then an attitude of denial on the part of the client will preclude its attainment, for the alcoholic who denies his condition will either continue to drink or be in a continual state of frustration because he knows he cannot drink without getting into trouble one way or another.

Staffing Patterns

Staffing patterns of alcoholism treatment facilities will vary from one unit to another, depending, in general, upon the types of services that are being offered. For example, an inpatient facility with a detoxification center would need to have medical and nursing personnel available around the clock. A post-detoxification treatment program may still have twenty-four-hour nursing service but with a physician available only "on call." Both types of treatment units should be served by one or more psychiatrists, particularly in a detoxification center. The value of psychiatric services, however, diminishes considerably in a post-detoxification treatment program. In other words, the ancillary function of the medical personnel and the nonmedical rehabilitation personnel does a flip-flop when the treatment shifts from detoxification to a type of didactic-psychological adjustment-inspirational program of recovery.

Alcoholism treatment services are characteristically located in a state hospital setting; in both private and public general hospitals; in "substance abuse"* centers or chemical dependency units which may be located in a general hospital or may function as an independent entity of its own; in halfway houses; and in outpatient facilities, such as state operated mental health clinics. Also, a large nationwide treatment program has been established by the Veterans Administration. According to the *APA Monitor* (Warren, 1972, p. 7), "currently 1,500 beds are available in special alcohol treatment units in forty-one VA hospitals across the country. An additional twenty-four new and expanded alcohol units have been recommended for funding in fiscal year 1973 which will provide two thousand beds. The VA plan now calls for the establishment of a total of eighty alcohol units through fiscal year 1974 which will provide three thousand beds." This article further notes that the treatment units vary in size from fifteen to about one hundred inpatient beds. Various treatment approaches are used in programs that range from three to twelve weeks, but generally a program would include group therapy, vocational guidance, reeducation, patient self-government, Antabuse®, and AA meetings. An emphasis is also placed on aftercare and follow-up. The treatment program involves the services of psychologists, psychiatrists, social workers, paraprofessional workers, recovered alcoholics, and chaplains.

Similar kinds of alcoholism programs have been established

---

* In addition to alcohol, substance abuse refers to the abuse of such drugs as marijuana, the hallucinogens, amphetamines, the barbiturates, hypnotics like Doriden®, drugs for pain such as codeine and Darvon®, tranquilizers such as Thorazine® and Compazine®, anti-anxiety drugs like Librium®, anti-depressants such as Tofranil® and Elavil®, and even compulsive eating.

in state hospital systems. For example, the program at East Louisiana State Hospital in Jackson encompasses twenty-one days.
During this time, patients are given vitamins and a diet high in
protein. Drugs are prescribed as needed, primarily for anxiety,
depression, and insomnia. Patients participate in group therapy
and individual counseling; they attend lectures and are shown
movies for didactic and educational purposes. Although the patients are strongly encouraged to attend the AA meetings that are
held on the unit, attendance is not required. Yet the program is
thought of as "AA oriented." Regarding the staff, medical responsibility is assumed by an assigned psychiatrist, of course,
but the overall program functions under the direction of nonmedical personnel. Services for the unit come from the chap-
laincy, psychology, social service, psychiatry, and nursing and attendant services. The unit, fondly referred to as "Colony 8," is
also served by counselors specializing in alcoholism; additionally,
vocational counseling is available to patients on a referral basis.

There is a relatively new treatment center that opened in October 1971, in Omaha, Nebraska. It is known as the Eppley Complex Chemical Dependency Unit (C.D.U.), and it operates within the structure of the Nebraska Methodist Hospital. During the
first two years of operation, between October 1971 and October
1973, there was a continuous growth at the Eppley C.D.U.
in terms of both the physical plant and numbers of patients and
staff. For example, during the first month of operation, the average daily census was only five patients, as compared to the
month of October 1973, when the average daily patient census
was forty-one. The total number of patients served during this
two-year period was about five hundred (Crooks, 1973).

Perhaps the best way to describe the program at Eppley C.D.U.
would be to outline the schedule of activities for the patients on
a typical day. Patients rise at 7:00 AM, make their beds, and otherwise get ready for breakfast, which is served at 8:00 AM. Between 8:30 and 9:00 AM various patient work details (such as
vacuuming the carpet, setting the dining room table, making
coffee, and keeping the TV lounge clean) are taken care of.
From 9:00 to 9:30 AM, patients either hear a didactic lecture on
topics ranging from the nature of alcoholism and drug addic-

tion to the twelve suggested steps of recovery in AA, or view a movie on alcoholism. Between 10:00 AM and 12:00 noon, patients participate in small group therapy sessions led by a staff counselor. Then, after lunch, there is another thirty minute lecture. From 2:00 to 5:00 PM, patients may be seen for individual counseling; they may be scheduled for an intake interview or for psychological testing (i.e. Minnesota Multiphasic Personality Inventory and Shipley-Hartford Test); a patient may be seen by his psychiatrist or by other physicians for medical problems. Patients may read, especially those books and pamphlets furnished by the counselors (e.g. the "big book" entitled *Alcoholics Anonymous, Twelve Steps and Twelve Traditions, Why Am I Afraid to Tell You Who I Am?, Your God Is Too Small*) or they may participate in certain leisure activities, such as playing cards, watching TV, or taking a walk in the park. Following the evening meal, patients attend AA meetings six nights a week held by a member of Alcoholics Anonymous who lives in the vicinity and oftentimes is a former patient of the unit.

The Eppley program is set up for about twenty-eight days. Following detoxification, the patient is assigned to a group and is also seen for individual counseling. Prior to being discharged, he must have completed the first five of the twelve steps of the AA recovery program. The first three steps are dealt with quite well in individual counseling and group therapy sessions, but step #4, "made a searching and fearless moral inventory of ourselves," must be completed alone. Step #5, "admitted to God, to ourselves, and to another human being the exact nature of our wrongs" (*Alcoholics Anonymous*, 1955, p. 59), must be taken in a one-to-one relationship with a chaplain who consults to the unit.

The unit also has an outpatient program similar to the daytime activities of the inpatients for the spouses and other family members of the alcoholic. Alcoholic patients are strongly encouraged to affiliate with an AA group of their own choosing after discharge and to work the remaining steps of the AA program. The non-alcoholic outpatients are urged to associate with Al-Anon.

In addition to the Director, staffing at the Eppley C.D.U. includes the gamut of medical and psychiatric consultants, round-the-clock registered nursing personnel, nurses' aides, a psychologist, a psychological examiner, five counselors, an average of about three counselors-in-training, and four consultant chaplains.

Among some of the other more recently established and highly regarded treatment facilities are the centers located in St. John's Hospital, St. Paul, Minnesota, Roosevelt Hospital, New York City, and Lutheran General Hospital, Park Ridge (near Chicago), Illinois. Hazelden Foundation, considered by some to be the granddaddy of the modern treatment programs for the alcoholic, is another well-recognized treatment facility and is located about forty miles from the St. Paul/Minneapolis area. The Roosevelt program operates in conjunction with the Columbia University Medical School and is patterned after the program at Hazelden (Smithers, 1972). In fact, the Eppley, C.D.U. program is also patterned after Hazelden. Lutheran General Hospital, according to Keller (1972), is a sixty-four-bed facility dedicated in 1969 for treatment, training, and research in alcoholism.

Cooperating Agencies and Professionals

In addition to the Vocational Rehabilitation Administration, other federal agencies such as the Community Services Branch of the National Institute on Alcohol Abuse and Alcoholism (N.I.A.A.A.) and the Law Enforcement Assistance Administration (L.E.A.A.) in the Department of Justice are geared to help state governments provide services to the alcoholic. For example, there is money available to state rehabilitation agencies for evaluation, training, and placement purposes. L.E.A.A. has funds for detoxification centers, and N.I.A.A.A. has monies for the planning of community services and direct service grants for the implementation of plans to establish community service centers, including staffing grants.

Other sources of help that come from tax supported agencies are the state operated mental health centers and clinics. Alcoholism outpatient clinics function as part of a statewide mental health program, and halfway houses are sometimes partially subsidized with vocational rehabilitation funds (Blackburn, 1973). Also, in certain states, the indigent alcoholic may be able to obtain necessary medical assistance under Title XIX of the Social Security Act (Mendelson, 1967).

Depending upon the size and purpose of the facility, as well as the availability of funds, such agencies may employ one or more of the following categories of professionals: alcoholism counselors and therapists, rehabilitation counselors, social workers, clinical and counseling psychologists, psychological examiners, registered and practical nurses, nurses aides, and psychiatrists and other physicians. We also find psychiatrists and other M.D.'s, psychologists, social workers, and counselors working with alcoholics in private practice or private psychiatric hospitals or clinics. Unfortunately, however, we cannot necessarily assume that all professionals who work with alcoholics have had appropriate training in the field of alcoholism. Some have and some have not. This situation is partially due to the recent influx of available jobs in the alcoholism field and the demand to fill open positions, which, in some cases, result in inadequately trained personnel rendering services that they are unqualified to handle. In other words, just because an individual is a clinical or counseling psychologist with an M.A. or Ph.D. degree or a psychiatrist with an M.D. degree or a social worker with an M.S.W. and an A.C.S.W., titles and degrees not automatically qualify a person to work competently with alcoholics. By the same token, it can be said (contrary to what some AA members believe) that just because a person is a sober (abstinent) alcoholic and a member of AA, this does not necessarily qualify him to work with efficacy with the practicing (still drinking) alcoholic. Yet there does appear to be certain professionals and paraprofessionals, in particular AA members, who without proper training possess the innate talent (presumably connected with the ability to empathize) to effectively work with the still suffering alcoholic.

The agency that is oftentimes the alcoholic's first contact prior to entering treatment or otherwise getting help for his problem is the local Council on Alcoholism. The function of a local council is to enlighten the public about the alcoholism problem and to refer clients, who may be either the alcoholic or members of the family of the alcoholic, to the proper source for whatever help that is needed. It is becoming a cliché that alcoholism is a family illness, but it is true. The rest of the family gets sick (emotionally) right along with the alcoholic. Local councils on alcoholism work cooperatively with the National Council on Alcoholism, a clearinghouse for the dissemination of information on alcoholism.

If the alcoholic is drinking, he may be referred by the counselor, at the local council on alcoholism, to a hospital for detoxification, followed by participation in a treatment program especially designed for alcoholics. During treatment he is usually made aware of the recovery program of Alcoholics Anonymous and advised to at least look into what AA has to offer after discharge. The emphasis on affiliation with AA following discharge will depend upon the background of the staff at the treatment center. If the alcoholic is dry, i.e. not drinking and not in need of detoxification, he may be referred directly to AA or an outpatient clinic or both. Non-alcoholic spouses and other adult members of the family may be referred to Al-Anon (teenage children to Alateen) and to an outpatient facility as well.

Perhaps the best way to briefly define what AA is would be to cite the preamble that is typically read at the beginning of each meeting.

> Alcoholics Anonymous is a fellowship of men and women who share their experience, strength and hope with each other that they may solve their common problem and help others to recover from alcoholism. The only requirement for membership is a desire to stop drinking. There are no dues or fees for AA membership; we are self-supporting through our own contributions. AA is not allied with any sect, denomination, politics, organization or institution; does not wish to engage in any controversy; neither endorses nor opposes any causes. Our primary purpose is to stay sober and help other alcoholics to achieve sobriety.
>
> (*The Grapevine*, November, 1973, p. 1)

A similar statement of the purpose of the Al-Anon Family Groups briefly describes its mission.

The Al-Anon program is essentially a personal reorientation process based on The Twelve Steps of Alcoholics Anonymous. The Al-Anon Family Groups make up a fellowship of men and women whose lives have been disturbed by another's compulsive drinking. The members share their experience, strength and hope with each other in a continuing effort to achieve serenity. The groups meet to discuss the problems created by alcoholism. It is an informal fellowship whose members try to uncover and discourage negative reactions. The meetings provide an atmosphere in which the members learn to recognize their own faulty attitudes which may be aggravating the family difficulties.

(Al-Anon Family Group Headquarters, Inc. 1971, vii)

From the point of view of the alcoholic as well as the alcoholism treatment center, the most accessible and inexpensive follow-up procedure is found in the recovery program of Alcoholics Anonymous. There are numerous AA groups located in large and small cities, towns, and hamlets all across the nation and in a number of foreign countries around the world. If there should happen not to be an AA group in the alcoholic's home town, though, a group is likely to be found in a town nearby. There are AA members who are quite willing to meet a new "prospect" at the door of an inpatient treatment facility as he is being discharged, or at his home, and accompany him to his first meeting.

REFERENCES

AA Grapevine. The Alcoholics Anonymous Grapevine, Inc., New York, November, 1973.

Al-Anon Family Group Headquarters: *The Dilemma of the Alcoholic Marriage*, revised expanded edition. Cornwall, Cornwall Press, 1971.

Anonymous. *Alcoholics Anonymous.* New York, Alcoholics Anonymous World Services, Inc., 1955.

Bacon, S. D.: Summer School of Alcohol Studies. Rutgers University, Alumni Institute, 1972.

Bell, A. H.: Measure for adjustment of the physically disabled. *Psychol Rep*, 21:773-778, 1967.

Bell, A. H.: Toward a theory of adjustment for the chronically disabled. A paper presented at the annual meeting of the Southwestern Psychological Association, St. Louis, Missouri, 1970.

Bell, A. H.: The Bell alcoholism scale of adjustment, a validity study. *Q J Stud Alcohol*, 31:965-967, 1970.

Bell, A. H., and Stickel, T. L.: Denial and independence of institutionalized clients as measured by the Bell disability scale. *Rehabilitation Research and Practice Review*, 2:49-53, 1971.

Bell, A. H. and Weingold, H. P.: Demographic profile of the alcoholic. Unpublished Study, East Louisiana State Hospital, Jackson, Louisiana, 1968.

Bell, A. H., Weingold, H. P., and Lachin, J. M.: Measuring adjustment in patients disabled with alcoholism. *Q J Stud Alcohol, 30*:634-639, 1969.

Blackburn, F. C.: Personal communication. Baker, Louisiana, 1973.

Crooks, W. H.: Personal communication, Eppley Complex Chemical Dependency Unit, Nebraska Methodist Hospital, Omaha, 1973.

Eaton, K. L.: Summer School of Alcohol Studies. Rutgers University, Alumni Institute, 1972.

Jellinek, E. M.: *The Disease Concept of Alcoholism*. New Haven, Hillhouse, 1960.

Keller, J. E.: Summer School of Alcohol Studies. Rutgers University, Alumni Institute, 1972.

Lawlis, G. F. and Rubin, S. E.: 16-PF study of personality patterns in alcoholics. *Q J Stud Alcohol, 32*:318-327, 1971.

Mendelson, J. H.: Alcohol and Alcoholism. Washington, D. C., U. S. Government Printing Office, 1967.

Schmidt, M.: World Health Organization, Technical Reports Series, *48*, 1952.

Smithers, R. B.: Summer School of Alcohol Studies. Rutgers University, Alumni Institute, 1972.

Warren, J. (ed.): V.A. expands services in drug abuse and alcoholism. *APA Monitor, 3*, July, 1972.

Weingold, H. P., Lachin, J. M., Bell, A. H., and Coxe, R. C.: Depression as a symptom of alcoholism: Search for a phenomenon. *J Abnorm Psychol*, 73:195-197, 1968.

Chapter 5

WORKING WITH THE CULTURALLY DIFFERENT DISABLED IN REHABILITATION FACILITIES

John G. Cull and Richard E. Hardy

Perhaps one of the least understood minority groups in our society is that of culturally different individuals who have suffered disability. When we think about how an individual will react to illness or disability, we can safely say that each person reacts according to what is characteristic for his own personality. For instance, the person who has in the past shown a strong need for dependence on others, who has shown that he cannot lead an independent life, will usually react in maybe an even more dependent fashion once disability is evident. The person who has been strongly independent and mature in his own adjustment to life in general probably will make an adequate or more than adequate adjustment to disability.

In order to be successful in working with this group of individuals, the facility administrator needs to understand the outstanding cluster of problems centered around the lack of understanding of the background and motivation of this type of individual. The facility staff needs to better understand the general cultural stockpile of the disadvantaged—his family togetherness, his reluctance to relocate, his acceptance of poverty as a way of life, his district of others and the various communication barriers which exist between the counselor and the client. Again, to be effective, the staff should be prepared to try to overcome some of the ignorance, apathy and resistance to the problems of the disadvantaged by the general public and the ultimate employers of this group of people.

Most counseling strategies and service programs have been developed for middle-class clientele. They were not developed for the public welfare recipient type of client. Counseling strategies work very smoothly and efficiently if there is an underlying motivation for success and if the client is able to forego short-range goals for long-range planning.

While values of poor persons seem to differ from those of the middle-class person, it should be remembered that these values do not differ in all respects. Persons living in poverty seem to have a strong orientation in the present and short-term perspectives rather than long-range planning and goals. In addition, there is a definite feeling of fatalism and the belief in chances; impulsiveness and a general inability to delay immediate gratification or make definite plans for the future. Also, there is a thinking process that could be termed much more concrete in character than abstract. There are general feelings of inferiority and an acceptance of authoritarianism. Therefore, when an individual who has lived in a poverty environment during the formative years of his growth and development becomes disabled, the reaction is generally substantially different from those who have been reared in a middle-class environment.

The pattern or culture of poverty is at times viewed as a causative factor in poverty and in other times as a result. In other words, general feelings and emotions resulting from impoverished conditions can either perpetuate the poverty or these same psychological feelings can be viewed as those consequences of the actual environmental conditions. The important question revolves around whether the environment causes the internal psychological makeup or whether the internal psychological makeup helps create the environmental state in which the individual lives. There are affirmative and negative answers to both questions and there is considerable overlap in any type of explanation which might attempt to give answers.

Poverty is a relative condition since it varies enormously from country to country and region to region. The subculture of poverty, however, in terms of the traits it seems to bring with it, transcends regional, racial, social, class and national differences. Of course there are definite variations among countries and over periods of time. It is a well-known fact that poverty in the nineteenth century was a much more tolerable state than poverty in the twentieth century.

It is important for those working with the disabled disadvantaged to show that they have confidence in these clients' abilities to improve themselves not only from the poverty condition, but also from the point of view of whatever handicap the individual may have. In a recent study by Rosenthal and Jacobson (1968), results indicated that teachers who were led to believe that certain lower class students could show unusual gains during the year actually brought about these gains in the children (the students for whom they held positive expectations).

Impact of Poverty on the Individual

Poverty very definitely constitutes one of the most persistent and critical problems of modern life. The factors associated with poverty and destitution influence the individual's feelings of self-worth, self-regard and general self-concept. When the self-concept is altered, the individual's behavior is altered. In other words, what a man thinks of himself determines to a great extent how he will behave in any given situation. Self-concept greatly influences the behavior an individual exhibits to others. Pockets of poverty, then, offer their own patterns and their own subcultures, and ways of behavior are determined by persons living within these pockets of poverty. In order for an individual to maintain the level of self-esteem he wishes to hold, he must be accepted by those persons who are important to him. The persons he knows within these pockets of poverty determine his life goals, meanings and social roles to a considerable degree. The individual identifies himself and gives status to his being according to the value system of those around him, especially those important others who also predetermine his present and future behavioral roles. This fact is important in understanding why many persons who live within these pockets of poverty in both our rural areas and our urban areas do not avail themselves of various programs and opportunities, and in general, the services of the rehabilitation counselor. These individuals have found their present identity, and any threat to their way of life represents a threat to their person. Proposed changes bring about great feelings of anxiety; while persons in poverty are unhappy about their fate, they do not have the strength to change what they have become. They do not have the immediate motivation to change the life pattern with which they are comfortable and that pattern of behavior through which they have found identity.

Few individuals are strong enough to make an identity change on their own, and changes within these pockets of destitution often must come through a total community development process. Persons can change as a group, once change has begun, easier than they can change as separate individuals. Change, then, within these pockets of destitution must come about within individuals in groups. It cannot be achieved just by moving people to new geographic areas or mounting new programs which are aimed at the individual and which put basic and primary responsibility on the individual.

In order for individuals or groups to change they must be somewhat dissatisfied with their present state and their present self-image. People in poverty as well as people in the middle class and higher classes vary in their satisfaction with their self-image, and this is why some are more susceptible to change than others. It is important for the professionals in the rehabilitation field to ask for opinions of persons living in poverty in order that they can evaluate the present conditions of these individuals' lives and see whether or not the individuals wish to change in their communities and in their individual physical environment. Many poverty stricken individuals have no idea that they can bring about change in their lives and most have given little thought to the possibility of improving living conditions. Rehabilitation workers must be cognizant of the fact that the most effective way to change people is to treat them in accordance with the status in life which they would like to achieve. If an individual is to change behavioral patterns, he must be treated in a different manner from that to which he is accustomed.

The staff of a facility concerned with the culturally disadvantaged and disabled disadvantaged should keep in mind that the economic system does not provide a sufficient number of employment opportunities in terms of available and appropriate jobs. There is a chronic depression among many poor persons resulting from inadequate occupational, educational, social and economic opportunity. This chronic depression is accentuated in our rural areas. This depression leads to a considerable lack of sufficient motivation for adjustment and achievement within the highly competitive society of the United States today. Various facts of life of the hard core jobless are interrelated and multiple. There is a high level of physical and mental deficiency, a low education level and poverty abounds. There is a general feeling of alienation, a lack of training and employment opportunity and severe racial and cultural problems.

Persons who live in the culture of poverty adapt to the conditions of that culture. The conditions and general culture of poverty perpetuates itself to its effects on children from generation to generation. It is believed that by the time children are six or seven they have taken on attitudes and values of their subculture, and they are not psychologically able to cope with the changing conditions and take advantage of various training and job opportunities which may occur later in life. If a break alone is offered to these individuals, it would soon be apparent that they were not favorably disposed toward the generosity. Measures to overcome their basic cultural, social and economic experiences must be included as a part of any social action program or rehabilitative program before positive change can be expected.

Moynihan (1968) has indicated that intensive family and personal rehabilitation must make up a major part of the war on impoverished conditions. He has said that increased opportunity for decent and well-paying jobs are simply not enough. Moynihan maintains that for an unspecified number of American poor, deprivation over a long period of time has caused such serious personality difficulties (personality structure problems) that these persons are psychologically unable to avail themselves of the various training and job opportunities which might be available to them. When these personality structure problems have a chronic or permanent disability superimposed upon them, the reaction to the disability is severe and often devastating.

Under the best of circumstances the integrity of the family constellation is severely tested when disability occurs; the integrity of the family is definitely threatened when disability occurs in poverty families. One very important characteristic of poverty families is that they are in constant crisis. It seems that no sooner is one crisis worked out than another takes its place. There is always the financial situation; there is always sickness; there is always the situation of the possibility of divorce due to increased stress; there is always crime and a lack of a safe living environment for the weaker members of the family structure; there is always the child in trouble, and there is always the possibility of the loss of employment. There is always the stress of insufficient nutrition and insufficient provision for activities and entertainment. When these deficiencies are superimposed upon a crisis situation in the family, such as disability, the psychological reaction to the disability by both family members and the disabled is heightened. These constant crises have the effect of draining all the energy from the family and its members. Such emotionality takes a high toll in terms of the overall ability of the family unit or of an individual within the family.

To a large portion of the newly disabled from the deprived environment, the newly acquired status of disability is merely one more in a long series of misfortunes which he has encountered. While those from more affluent backgrounds are concerned about the future impact of the disability, those from the ghetto areas are more concerned with the here and now aspects of the disability.

When an individual accepts that his disability is of a permanent nature and that it is irrevocable, there will then be a period of what can be called reactive depression and, depending upon the severity of the disability, there may be various suicidal inclinations. This period of extreme depression after severe injury is a normal phase of adjustment. It is at this time that often much harm is done by well-meaning individuals who offer too much hope in terms of what may or may not be accomplished by science in order to aid the individual in the future. This is a period when candid advice and information can be of great value to the individual in planning what he is able to do in reference to his particular circumstance.

Accepting disability is of paramount importance. Persons vary in their reactions to a disability. Some think they are being punished for their own or for their parents' sins. Others may give the disability societal meaning in terms of their never being full members again with equal status. Still others may put sexual meanings on the disability problems. In addition, the economic aspect of the problem is often emphasized.

The meaning of disability to the family and friends of the individual cannot be overly stressed. If a child, for instance, is born disabled, the family is not only grief stricken, but since the child represents the family's position in the community, the disabled child is more than a disappointment. Often the families of these children can find little happiness in caring for them. Often they enter upon every expensive endeavor to ameliorate a disability which cannot be corrected. In some cases the father will completely abandon the disabled child and his family saying that the defective child is the mother's responsibility since she gave birth to it. The family often can disintegrate around arguments and disputes which center around a disabled child.

Special Problems in Adolescence

There are important reasons why traumatic experiences during adolescence can be of particular significance to the individual. Physique plays an especially important part in how we look at ourselves and in adolescence the body is constantly changing. In addition, the adolescent period overlaps both childhood and adulthood, and it is during the period of adolescence that important self-concept changes take place. During this period an individual is making a real effort to get to know himself, his abilities, and his limitations. If traumatic injury causes disability during this period, the adjustment to such disability can be of extreme difficulty.

During adolescence, the young person is particularly concerned about his physique in terms of sexuality. The young person is very interested in learning how others will view him from the point of view of his sexual role. He has constantly heard about marriage and bearing offspring and is evaluating how he will measure up to the criteria established by society. The adolescent who sustains a disability must tolerate the frustration and psychological meaning to him as an individual of this disability plus the overlapping child-adult status which he holds. The fact that he is disabled may cause the overlapping of childhood and adulthood to persist into years beyond that of the usual adolescent period. When the person is denied adulthood status due to disability which may retard his forward movement, insecurities increase. It should be noted that the tremendous influence of the adolescent's peer group during this period has a great deal to do with how he evaluates himself in comparison with what he would like to be later as an adult. It is easy for the adolescent during this difficult period to develop contempt for adult authority and to become very cynical even without the added burden of a disabling circumstance.

Slums offer their own patterns and their own subcultures. Their ways of behavior are determined by persons living within them. In order for an individual to maintain the level of self-esteem he wishes to hold, he must be accepted by those persons who are important to him within his environment. The persons he knows within the slums or ghetto determine life goals, meanings, and social roles for him to a considerable degree. It is of prime importance for him to be accepted by them and be accepted by himself at the same time. The individual identifies himself and gives status to his *being* according to the values of those around him, especially to those important *others* who almost predetermine his present and future behavior and goals. This fact is important in understanding why many persons who live within the ghetto and within slums do not avail themselves of various training and placement opportunities and in general, the services of the rehabilitation counselor. These individuals have found their present identity and any threat to their way of life represents a threat to their person. Proposed changes by the rehabilitation counselor bring about great feelings of anxiety. While persons in poverty are unhappy with their fate, they do not have the strength to change that which they have become comfortable with and that pattern of behavior through which they have found identity. Consequently, in the face of the onset of disability, it is much more likely that the individual will seek to achieve a level of adjustment in the environment in which he lives which existed prior to the onset of disability than strike out in a new area and achieve at a higher level even though he may be fully capable intellectually and vocationally to accomplish at a higher level. The problem here is that disability had added an additional stress in the equilibrium he has established between his own personality integration and the demands and stress of the environment. The psychological adjustment to disability among poverty groups is most difficult with individuals in early adolescence up through early adulthood since they are adjusting to a life-style which makes unusual and somewhat severe psychological demands upon them thereby reducing the available psychic reserves to adjust to other conditions.

Few individuals are strong enough to make an identity change on their own and changes within areas of the ghetto and slum often much come through a total community development process. Persons can change once change has begun easier than they can change on their own initiative as separate individuals. Change then within slums and ghettos must come about within individuals and groups and cannot be achieved just by moving people to new geographical areas and physical surroundings and providing rehabilitation services in these new surroundings.

In order for disabled individuals to change they must be somewhat dissatisfied with their present state—their present self-image. Disabled people in poverty, as well as people in middle and higher classes, vary in their satisfaction with their self-image and this is why some are more susceptible to change than others. This is why some are more receptive to counseling services than others. It is important for social service workers to ask for opinions of the disabled living in poverty in order that they can evaluate the present conditions of these individuals' lives and see whether or not they wish to change in their communities and in their individual physical environments. Many of these people have no idea that they could bring about a change in their lives and have given little thought to the possibilities of improving their living conditions. The concept of vocational rehabilitation in many of these instances is totally alien and incompatible with their life style. Those working with the disabled in these areas must be cognizant of the fact that the most effective way to change people is to treat them in accordance with the status in life which they would like to achieve. If an individual is to change behavioral patterns he must be treated or rewarded in a manner different from that to which he is accustomed.

Implications for Counselors in Facilities

Now, based upon this pattern, the counselors within our communities will be challenged in working with this large segment of our population. Old approaches will no longer work. Counselors who do not tool up and modify their basic approaches in evaluating clients and providing counseling services will be left behind during the mid and later seventies when the clamor for welfare reform will reach its peak. Not only must we work with the individual as we have in the past, but we must now work with his family in a more intimate and dramatic fashion. We must work with other community organizations which are organized for meeting some of the clients' needs. Additionally, we must work with the client in different program approaches and different counseling approaches than we have recognized in the past.

In working with the disadvantaged, it is clearly indicated that different counseling approaches will need to be developed. Some old counseling strategies may be modified for the particular needs of this segment of our culture, but we feel new levels of involvement need to be developed and new counseling strategies need to emerge in order to adequately meet counseling needs of this population. The counselor will need to work more closely with the community to learn how to uncover community resources, to work with family members, and to deal with the basic problems of transportation, housing, and food supplement. Concepts such as self-actualization and client self-direction should not be ignored, but emphasis in the counseling strategy must be upon meeting current emergencies. With this approach self-direction and other long-range goals may eventually become a meaningful reality to the client; however, they should not be interjected as early in the process as they have been in the past. This is a quite obvious conclusion when one considers the level of our clients in the past in relationship to Maslow's Hierarchy (Maslow, 1954). According to Maslow's Hierarchy, most of our clients in the past have fulfilled the specific needs at the most basic two levels and are involved in fulfilling love and esteem needs. This new segment of clients with which we will be dealing are concerned more with physiological needs and safety needs. Therefore, their concerns are much more immediate and much more urgent.

Basic security in coping with the environment and with immediate concerns and problems are paramount values of the disadvantaged. Planning ahead is often a futile exercise and holds little personal value or rewards. For example, the possibility of discontinuance of a basic income supplement through a Social Security pension or welfare is apt to be viewed negatively in light of previous limited job success and long periods of unemployment frustration. Such clients have little assurance that social services, counseling, and rehabilitation will make them better off than they are now.

An important problem affecting the counseling outcome is that the client may feel counselors really do not understand him or his needs; furthermore, he may feel that the team members working in the rehabilitation process may try to convey the attitude of understanding, but from the client's viewpoint, these individuals really do not and cannot understand. For example, the client will agree that personal motivation is necessary for people to get ahead in the world; however, the client is apt to disagree seriously if the counselor questions the client's motivation. The need for immediate assistance, medical care, transportation, and money are seen as the most important first steps. Many people needing the services of rehabilitation counseling feel they previously have been given unfulfilled promises by the professional personnel in the various fields of social service. There are psychological needs requiring immediate reward or service. Long-term planning and vague expectations and promises fail to motivate most disabled disadvantaged people.

Furthermore, a client has a general pessimism which is hard for the highly goal-oriented, motivated professionals to understand. The client has seen few of his people make it. Those who have escaped from poverty seldom remain in his social group, and hence, are not present to serve as models with whom the client might identify. Thus, the things which the client considers to be important are not apt to be congruent with what the counselor considers to be of importance.

In light of these considerations, perhaps now it can be understood why a client may drop a training program, which could eventually lead to a two or three dollar an hour job, for an immediate opportunity to accept a job paying $1.50 per hour. Such behavior is understandable even though it appears to us to be a dead-end and self-defeating action.

The client desperately needs to be considered important and may really want to feel that he is being accepted by professionals working with him; yet, many clients may have had previous experience with public agencies when they felt that their own personal integrity was questioned and their experience with the agency was a personally degrading one. Thus, they are now apt to view the counselor with suspicion and he must be proven not guilty. Demonstrating and conveying instant acceptance of the client as a worthwhile individual is a first major step toward establishing a working relationship.

The counselor has a prime opportunity to serve in a very basic capacity; he should be the focal point of community action and rehabilitation services. The counselor should serve not only as a focal point but as an energizer of services. There is a common concept that there is a paucity or a lacking of services within our communities organized to meet the needs of this segment of our population. This is not true. Upon investigation, one will find a plethora of services, however, they tend to be somewhat disjointed and directed more toward specific groups of people. Quite often their approach is less broad than we would desire. Therefore, the counselor should assume the role of being the uniting force between these diverse service agencies for the benefit of these disadvantaged disabled clients. He should develop a very active information and referral program in order to be able to know who is providing services to what groups, where the clientele are located and what their needs are. In order to serve the welfare recipient, we have to find him. If the rehabilitation counselor is not able to locate and identify concentrations of welfare recipient clients, he cannot serve as an effective ingredient in the rehabilitation process.

Therefore, it would behoove the counselor to take time to learn each agency's function and solicit its cooperation. In order for the counselor to achieve the bright promise which lies ahead in fulfilling his role in the rehabilitation of this segment of our population, he should become a force in welding the community together and directing it toward this goal.

Since communicating with the public welfare recipient is a prime obstacle to successful rehabilitation, we feel the counselor should initiate the employment of indigenous workers to communicate with these clients. The indigenous worker who is carefully selected to work with his people can do much more in the way of communicating to these citizens in bringing about the necessary changes that are indicated in order for the client to be employed than can a professional worker in many cases.

Since there is a shortage of available manpower within our professional areas, we need to turn to innovative approaches in staffing patterns. One innovative approach is the use of volunteer workers. We have a large reservoir of untapped manpower within the retired ranks of our communities. We feel the rehabilitation facilities within the country have missed the boat by not mobilizing these people for rehabilitation purposes. We have seen evidence that retired people from all walks of life are interested in volunteering their services to rehabilitation facilities. We have seen demonstrated that these individuals are eager to accept responsibility for the transportation of clients to rehabilitation facilities, clinics and various other facilities. We have seen clients who are eager to accept responsibility in functioning as remedial educators for clients who are in need of remedial education; we have seen retired individuals who will volunteer to work with clients who are involved in homebound programs. It is our opinion that the counselor should make maximum utilization of voluntary activity.

REFERENCES

Cull, J. G., and Hardy, R. E.: *Rehabilitation of the Urban Disadvantaged.* Thomas, Springfield, 1973.

Hardy, R. E. and Cull, J. G.: *Climbing Ghetto Walls.* Thomas, Springfield, 1973.

Maslow, A. H.: *Motivation and Personality.* New York, Harper & Row, 1954.

Moynihan, D. P.: *Maximum Feasible Misunderstanding.* New York, Free Press, 1968.

Rosenthal, R. and Jacobson, L. F.: Teacher expectations for the disadvantaged. *Sci Am, 218*:19-23, 1968.

CHAPTER 6

SERVING THE PUBLIC OFFENDER IN REHABILITATION FACILITIES

DENNIS A. GAY

FACILITIES FOR PUBLIC offenders have existed for centuries in nearly every known culture. Facilities for helping the public offender become a useful contributing member of society, however, are relatively new to the scene, and are entangled in much controversy, political and otherwise, the issue of retribution vs. rehabilitation. Because 95 percent of incarcerated public offenders eventually return to society, most within a relatively short period of time, and since for the most part prisons do little more than increase the problems of the public offender and subsequently the problems of society, there has been increased interest in alternate approaches to the problems of the public offender. Some of these approaches are reflected in current trends in the courts and correctional systems, e.g.: an increased number of convictions resulting in probation rather than institutional placement, more lenient sentences given for first or second offenses, and for the lesser offenses, increased efforts toward rehabilitation within the correctional institution, as well as providing rehabilitation services outside the institution in the way of halfway houses, workshops, and rehabilitation facilities.

Because the scope of facilities intended for serving the public offender is such a broad one, ranging from small treatment units in prisons to large elaborate facilities designed to deal with all phases of the individual's life, the following discussion is an attempt to select those aspects of serving the public offender in a rehabilitation facility which are the most common to facilities in general and, hopefully, of the most concern and benefit to practitioners working with or within a rehabilitation-oriented facility. An introduction and discussion of some of the most commonly observed characteristics of this client group is followed by general considerations of initial intake, evaluation and program planning, the provision of services, and the termination of services.

Who Is the Public Offender?

Nearly everyone, when asked, will admit to having committed public offenses of some sort; the chances are good that at some time, in some state, the offense committed is considered a felony which could have brought a jail or prison sentence. Delinquent and criminal acts are committed quite regularly by people at all levels of society, but the majority of the people committing these acts are not identified as public offenders, at least not in the sense of needing some form of rehabilitation service. Who then is the public offender who concerns social service and correctional workers? Maybe what is really being asked is who is in our prisons, or who is most likely to be referred for rehabilitation services?

Biographical Aspects

A basic profile can be assembled, although it must be kept in mind that some public offenders do not fit into all, or even any, of the categories. The profile is very general and can best be described as a composite of the most commonly observed characteristics.

The *typical* public offender comes from the lower or lower-middle socioeconomic class and more than likely has lived in some form of deprivation. He is male (eight men to every woman) and may very well be a member of a minority group, usually black or Chicano. (Although there are more whites incarcerated across the country, percentagewise there are more minority members in our prisons.) The probability is very high that he is single, and if married, the chances are great that there is considerable marital and family difficulty. Marital problems are closely associated with other problems of the public offender and it is rare that a marriage and family will hold together through most of the difficulties a public offender experiences, particularly incarceration. This should not imply that family ties are not important to the public offender. Danial Glasser (1964) suggests that along with a good job, a good woman is probably the best step toward rehabilitation. In his pattern of inadequate behaviors lie the offender's inability to maintain a sound marital relationship.

The mobility of the public offender far exceeds that of the general population. This of course is related to his general overall pattern of instability. He tends to change jobs, addresses, cities, and even states quite frequently. This factor can cause considerable problems for the rehabilitation worker and often leads to general discouragement. The public offender will more than likely have serious educational deficiencies, and will have probably completed less than the eighth grade. Although a large number of offenders have been considered retarded because of low IQ scores, the overall profile is quite similar to the general population.

Psychological Aspects

The psychological patterns of the typical public offender are not those of the textbook psychopath, though he may have some personality traits associated with psychopathy. The personality traits observed most often are hostility, impatience, anxiety, manipulation, a need for immediate gratification, and a need to express bravado and manliness. The hostility may be covert initially and directed toward many objects including the establishment, society, self, family, and authority figures in general. The manipulative behavior, along with hostility, apparent selfishness, and the immature need for immediate gratification which is observed in so many public offenders, has led to the label of sociopath. This label, as with other labels, is usually unnecessary and in some instances detrimental. When one considers that the American Psychiatric Association (1968) has some twenty odd categories dealing with behavior disorders, the complexity of the issue can be recognized.

The characteristics discussed vary in degree when one works with individuals. The rehabilitation worker will encounter a wide spectrum of behavior patterns in the clients with whom he works, ranging from simple, immature, inadequate behavior to more ingrained character disorders. It is unlikely that the rehabilitation facility will be adequately equipped to work with the more serious forms of psychoses sometimes encountered in public offenders, and it should be attempted only under adequate medical supervision.

Legal Aspects

Rehabilitation workers not directly connected with a correctional institution are often confused by the legal status assigned to their clients. It should be helpful, therefore, to discuss these aspects at this point.

The legal status of juveniles has always been confusing and more complicated than that of adults. This was particularly true prior to the 1967 *Gault* decision* which has prompted a series of revisions of juvenile codes in many states across the nation. In general, states follow a scheme whereby children under the age of sixteen are dealt with in juvenile courts only and juveniles between sixteen and eighteen may be tried in either juvenile or adult court depending upon certain factors including the severity of the offense. Usually persons over the age of eighteen are considered adults and tried in adult courts. If the court so decides, the juvenile court may take custody of the child. He may receive probation or be placed in an institution and later remain under supervision for a period of time after release. In the past, indefinite sentences up to age twenty-one were very common with juveniles.

The legal status of the adult offender is more definitive. At the point of conviction, the parole and probation department usually becomes involved and a sentence is later handed down. If the offender is placed on probation, it is in lieu of incarceration and he will not be sent to an institution unless dealt with for some infraction (revoked). He will instead be under the supervision of a probation officer for a specified period of time. In the event the sentence calls for incarceration, the person will be placed in an institution and eventually, with the exception of rare cases, return to a community on parole. He will then remain under

---

* For a complete discussion of the *Gault v. Arizona* Supreme Court Decision, the reader is referred to: Nordin, Virginia D. (Ed.): *Gault: What Now for the Juvenile Court.* Ann Arbor, Institute of Continuing Legal Education, 1968.

parole supervision for a specified period of time relating to his original sentence. Very briefly, *probation* is in lieu of going to an institution, and *parole* is a privilege allowed whereby an offender who has been in an institution is allowed to finish out his sentence under supervision in the community.

It is seldom that a rehabilitation worker will find himself working with a public offender, who is not under the supervision of either an institution, as in the case of special "work-release" programs, or of the probation or parole agency. Because of this, the first concern should be to establish contact with the supervising agent and begin a coordinating effort.

Intake

Most rehabilitation facilities are not required by law to accept all referrals as clients, and it is therefore necessary for them to establish policies regarding intake.

Intake policies necessarily vary from facility to facility, and there should not be a single policy which is forced to fit all facilities. However, a number of guidelines have proven helpful when working with the public offender and are discussed here under the headings of selection and stabilization.

Selection

The selection of clients into the program is probably the most important single key to the success or failure of the client. A facility should not accept the more difficult public offender clients unless it is geared up to deal with the types of problems that ensue. When a client is accepted into a program and is later terminated because of problems, it constitutes "one more failure" for the client, and a great many public offenders have known little else but failure all of their lives. It is the facility's responsibility to insure that when failure occurs, it is not because of poor judgment on the part of the staff in terms of unrealistic thinking.

It sometimes happens that correctional personnel or vocational rehabilitation counselors will, out of desperation, refer clients who have a very poor prognosis for rehabilitation.

Even though the rehabilitation workers are trying to do the best job possible, the facility worker must be careful not to fill his program with extremely difficult cases and later find that he is unable to be effective with anyone because of the multitude of problems. This is not to imply that chances should never be taken in the interest of a client with a poor prognosis for rehabilitation. Judgment, however, is important in terms of keeping the number and difficulty of the cases within the realistic boundaries of the facility's resources.

Prior to actual acceptance of a client into the program, the facility worker should hold an in-depth interview with all parties directly involved. There will usually be the correctional worker (most often a parole officer, probation officer or institutional caseworker) the sponsoring agency representative (often a vocational rehabilitation counselor) and the client. As a result of these interviews, information relevant to the client's feasibility for the program should be gathered from the client's background and current status. Special attention should be given to the home and/or family situation. Experience has shown that home and family environmental factors tend to be closely correlated to the client's ability and willingness to accept services and his eventual successful rehabilitation. In addition, it has been found that personality characteristics tend to be more important determinants of success in public offenders than are intelligence, interests, or aptitudes.

Lastly, prior to final acceptance, two more guidelines will prove very helpful. The first is the establishment of a regular system of communication with the other parties involved for purposes of progress reports and any other assistance they can provide. Quite often attendance problems can be precluded by a mutual agreement established with the assistance of the other parties prior to acceptance.

The last recommendation relating to selection is that a firm commitment be made on the part of the client to participate in the program. Very often programs in corrections are set up for clients according to what everyone else involved wants for the client with little or no attention given to what the client really wants. Even when the client agrees to become involved in a program, it is sometimes difficult to ascertain whether he is genuinely interested or succumbing to various pressures. An in-depth interview with the client can often detect the true situation. At other times, the client simply does not know what he wants and a firm commitment from the client to give the program a fair chance can be very important.

Public offenders have acquired the reputation of being very manipulative, and as a result many rehabilitation workers are hesitant to become involved with them for fear of being manipulated. They view manipulation as akin to "being made a fool of." Manipulation most certainly will exist, but it is not necessarily always bad, for it at least indicates that the individual is trying to help himself, which can be a good start. A worker who is aware of manipulation and who has the skill and patience to deal with it can often help the client channel the manipulation energy into more constructive methods of dealing with his environment. Manipulation can sometimes be healthy and positive. However, when it is used to put other people down or to point out what *suckers* others are, it becomes unhealthy and negative.

Stabilization

The initial stabilization of the public offender's life situation becomes a very important part of the facility's intake process when the client has just recently been released from jail, prison, or has just undergone some crisis situation. A public offender coming to a rehabilitation facility will very likely be in one of these categories. It is not uncommon for the public offender to enter into one crisis after another, either emotionally or otherwise. And very often a problem in one area of his life will affect all the other areas. For example, if a marriage or love affair goes sour, he may lose his job, quit a training program, commit another offense, or abscond from supervision. A lack of tolerance for even the slightest disappointment is often present and can be responsible for yet another failure.

Most authorities agree that the first thirty to sixty days after release from an institution are the most crucial for rehabilitation intervention. When a public offender returns to the community, he is usually very unsettled and anxious about any number of problems, such as his family, his job situation, living arrangements, and transportation. For this reason, it is very important that he be somewhat settled before entering the rehabilitation facility, unless, of course, the facility is of the "live-in" type. Then, some of the problems are already solved. However, most facilities are not able to provide for housing, transportation, and living expenses. Vocational rehabilitation counselors and parole or probation officers can help in this respect. However, the size of caseloads in both of these agencies is usually very large and clients often do not get all the attention they require. The facility worker should be prepared to spend a good deal of time assisting and coordinating the stabilization effort in the early phases of intake. Not only will this help the client through a difficult period, but it will provide an opportunity for a closer relationship between the facility worker and the client, thus helping to lay the groundwork for a more successful beginning.

Evaluation and Planning

Much of the evaluation and planning process will have already begun as a result of information gathered for intake purposes. However, more will have to be done in order to better understand the problems the client is facing to assist him in his medical, social and vocational goals.

The possibility of medical problems should not be overlooked in an evaluation. Although the majority of public offenders will become clients of a rehabilitation facility because of a history of behavior problems, a complete medical examination will sometimes reveal a medical problem which has escaped detection or has been minimized in the past. Hidden disabilities, such as diabetes or other system imbalances in addition to poor vision or hearing, have been known to affect an individual's behavior to a marked degree. Sometimes medical assistance can eliminate a good many problems. If the only medical information is skimpy or outdated, the facility should request a more recent examination.

Social and Psychological Evaluation

Social and psychological evaluations for public offenders are procured in much the same way as the more traditional client's evaluation, with the possible exception of more emphasis placed on direct observation and interview as opposed to paper and pencil tests only. A good deal of the social history material has already been compiled by the corrections workers and can be helpful when interviewing the client. When feasible, family and other persons close to the client should be included in the evaluation, as well as in later phases of the program.

As mentioned previously, psychological factors and personality characteristics play an important part in the evaluation process and have considerable bearing on the outcome of services. It is therefore useful to devise a number of situational evaluations in addition to the usual psychological instruments. Efforts should be made to observe the client in a number of different settings. Does he function better alone, or with others in a group? Is he shy? Who does he get along with best? How does he ventilate his anger? Does he keep it bottled up inside? Very often this kind of direct observation produces much more helpful information than do tests. The problem, of course, is that this requires not only a good deal of time and effort on the part of the facility, but also requires the facility to be large enough to offer a number of different situations for observation.

If the client is observed to be manipulative of staff and other clients, it should be pointed out and plans made for confrontation with the client through counseling and other methods.

Vocational Evaluation and Planning

The vocational aspects of a public offender's life are very important and usually in need of considerable attention. If a public offender is functioning adequately in a good job, it is usually an indication that other aspects of his life are going pretty well also. Employment stability or the lack of it, has been shown time and again to be an important prediction of recidivism (returning to prison) or eventual rehabilitation. For this reason, the vocational evaluation should constitute a major portion of the program in a rehabilitation facility.

Background information and the work history interview are first steps in vocational appraisal. Careful interviews should be conducted with some time spent exploring avocational interests as well as vocational. Avocational pursuits can often offer clues to specific interests and skills that the client himself has not considered.

In addition to the standard paper and pencil tests for interests, achievement, and abilities, a number of work tasks can be developed or purchased by the facility. As in the case of the social and psychological evaluation, direct observation on a number of various tasks is a supplement to vocational testing. Work assignments can be used in this way as well. The client should be re-evaluated frequently with regard to such factors as level of functioning, motivation, work habits, attitudes, and interpersonal relations.

Casual discussions with the client's caseworker and the perceptions of the various staff who have the opportunity to observe the client over a period of time are valuable sources of information. It will be interesting to discover how different people observe the same person in different situations.

Unfortunately, many correctional institutions and some rehabilitation facilities are equipped to provide work evaluation and training in only those areas which directly benefit the institution or facility. Examples of these trades are barbers, cooks, bakers, kitchen helpers, laundry workers, janitors, and shoe repairmen, all of which need to be done in the everyday operation of the institution. While careful and honest use of these jobs can provide useful evaluation and training, the danger of misuse in terms of placing more emphasis on getting the jobs done for the sake of the institution and less emphasis on a meaningful evaluation or training experience is always present.

Vocational evaluation and planning with public offender clients is not an easy task, and care must be taken against hasty judgments which lead to eventual failure. It is not enough to find something the client can do. As people with experience in corrections will testify; it is relatively easy for most public offenders to find a job. The problem lies in their keeping a job for a substantial period of time.

Evaluation and planning needs to be a comprehensive cooperative effort. Social, familial, and psychological factors require consideration in vocational evaluation and planning for public offenders even more than with traditional physically disabled clients, because the public offender's problems are so often related to these areas.

Realistic vocational goals are a major problem among the younger public offender clients, in particular, and considerable time needs to be spent along these lines. The younger males seem to prefer the masculine stereotyped jobs which pay big money: heavy equipment operators, long-haul truck drivers, or diesel mechanics; the younger females prefer the glamorous jobs such as cosmetologist or model. Certainly these vocations should not be ruled out without consideration; the competition, however, is extremely keen in these areas, and the feasibility for a large number of clients is doubtful.

It seems appropriate at this point to provide three recommendations regarding vocational planning which elicit enough consensus among experienced workers in the field to warrant their review:

a. *Avoid finalizing the rehabilitation plan while the client is still incarcerated.* The rehabilitation worker must realize that goals developed while clients are institutionalized are frequently modified or abandoned soon after release. Many goals are based on fantasy or are hastily contrived to persuade parole boards and other authorities that the client is ready for release. The majority of his mental energy, while he is incarcerated, is quite naturally directed toward getting out as soon as possible. This overriding preoccupation very often produces unrealistic and unachievable goals.

b. *Avoid long-term training programs in favor of on-the-job training or short-term vocational training.* Vocational training is often a very necessary and desirable plan for public offender clients. However, long-term training has all too frequently resulted in failure because of the immediate needs of the client and his inability to persevere without quick tangible results. Also, in some cases where successful college training has resulted, the degree was in an area of relatively no use to the client in terms of a job. Some examples are degrees in history, music, art, psychology, sociology, and political science, as a B.A. or B.S. in these fields are often useless except for entrance into graduate school.

c. *Avoid small business ventures.* Periodically the worker will encounter a client who has a special talent in shoe repairing, tailoring (leather or textile), cooking, baking, crafting, or auto mechanics, and who has a desire to get into business for himself. He may even have been in business in the past. These business plans have been attempted many times, and as a general rule have proven to be a very expensive lesson for the sponsoring agency. Small businesses are notorious for failing even under the most optimal conditions.

While the above recommendations appear to be in a rather negative tone, they should not be taken as such. The primary task of the rehabilitation worker is to help provide "successes" for his client, not more failures. These recommendations are simply drawing attention to high failure probability plans.

The importance of coordinating all efforts with participating agencies cannot be stressed too heavily. This is particularly true of the corrections agency involved. The corrections agent has legal responsibility for the supervision of his client and therefore must approve any conditions or plans suggested by the facility. Correctional workers are more than happy to get all the help they can, particularly if they feel the facility will benefit their client and keep him out of trouble.

Rehabilitation Services

Some rehabilitation facilities are large enough to provide a wide range of services to their clients, including psychotherapy, medical therapy, training in a wide variety of skills, eventual job placement, and follow-up for a period of time after the client is working. Other facilities are able to provide only evaluation and planning as a service. Regardless of the scope of services provided by a facility, counseling and some type of training are offered by most facilities and are worthy of some attention in serving the public offender.

Counseling the Public Offender

Counseling public offenders requires all of the skills necessary for counseling in general and more. Certain personality traits and subsequent behaviors common to this group of clients can be overbearing at times even to the experienced counselor. The counselor often feels unappreciated, ineffective and generally frustrated after having spent long hours and a great deal of effort trying to help a client who is not showing any improvement and, what is worse, does not seem to care. How far should I have to go to make someone want to help himself? Why should I have to put up with all of this when there are other clients I can work with who will appreciate me? These are typical questions a counselor working with public offenders will ask himself sooner or later. They are asked because the counselor is experiencing a personal affront to his own self-concept, or as psychoanalysts would explain, he is becoming ego-involved and his ego is threatened. It is the ability of the counselor to deal with this ego-involvement, or to "keep his cool" if you will, that constitutes the "more" that is required to effectively counsel the public offender.

Why are public offenders so difficult to work with? The answer is that all are not. But frequently clients with behavior disorder characteristics are very difficult to counsel. One theory suggests that interpersonal relationships have been failures for the client since early childhood. Every time he put his faith into a relationship, "stuck his neck out," so to speak, he was rejected in one way or another. Eventually he learned to play it safe, taking the negative approach, in this way not succumbing to failure. Later, when a counselor attempts to develop a relationship, the client is suspicious, uncooperative and even hostile, thus protecting himself against another failure. It will take much dedication, patience, perseverance and genuine interest on the part of the counselor to overcome this syndrome.

The counseling process actually begins at the intake stage and will continue throughout the client's contact with the facility. It should be a dynamic continuous process, devoid of moralizing, and should not be limited to the magic fifty minutes across the desk.

The counselor should get out of his office whenever possible and get involved with his client in various areas around the facility or outside the facility. Effective counseling can occur in a number of places such as in the work setting, over lunch, or just going for a walk. Effective counseling will require a genuine concern and willingness to take the kinds of personal risks discussed by Stratten (1973). He promotes "opening up" to another person without regard to loss of status, or the "personal risk that takes basic honesty, caring and warmth."

Most counselors agree that the amount of investment on the part of the counselor exceeds the returns to a much greater degree when counseling public offenders than is the case with other client groups. This should be understood by the counselor from the outset. He should not expect the client to "get well" and change his whole pattern of life functioning in a short period of time. Positive changes will be slight and slow in coming; there will be crises and major set-backs which will test the counselor's sincerity and ability. On occasion, there will be deliberate attempts on the part of the client to destroy the relationship that has been established.

The failure of counselors and other rehabilitation workers to cope with the problems presented by public offender clients is very often traced to the initial mental approach. If one approaches the job at hand with his mind set that problems should not exist, he can become extremely frustrated and discouraged when they inevitably occur. On the other hand, if one approaches the job knowing problems will occur, the frustration is lessened and he may have more energy to deal with them in a positive way.

Group counseling can be very effective with the public offender client under controlled conditions. The success of the group approach is directly related to the knowledge, training and ability of the group leader, in addition to the initial selection of the group members. Groups should be organized with specific purposes in mind, and the composition and organization of the group will be dependent upon its purpose. Groups may be organized for purposes of vocational orientation and adjustment, social and personal adjustment, or for psychotherapy, in which case a qualified clinical psychologist or psychiatrist should be involved.

Training in a Rehabilitation Facility

Vocational training is one of the earliest and probably still one of the most promising approaches toward rehabilitation of the public offender, provided it is adequate and appropriate and backed up by a broad spectrum of social and other supportive services. Unfortunately, the type and adequacy of training in correctional institutions and most rehabilitation facilities is limited drastically by space and funds. Prisons have been relatively unsuccessful in training inmates for competitive labor for a number of reasons. One is that the type of training is usually limited to the needs of the institution, which are often quite different from the needs of the outside world, and another is that even in the more promising training programs such as auto mechanics, electronics, and refrigeration, the level of proficiency acquired by the trainee is not high enough to make him competitive in the open market.

The following recommendations for rehabilitation facilities serving the public offender should prove helpful:

1. With respect to vocational course offerings, select training programs on the basis of high potential for actual employment. Not only should the demand for the skill be determined, but also the legal aspects pertaining to persons with prison records, since in some localities public offenders may be denied a barber's or driver's license, or be barred from jobs in hotels and restaurants.

2. With respect to course content, the level of proficiency required for competitive employment should be determined and integrated accordingly. A trainee in auto mechanics for example, will need to know much more today than was required just a few years ago. He should have a thorough knowledge of the more sophisticated pieces of electronic equipment presently used for tuning and troubleshooting. Similarly, the field of electronics is far advanced over the

electron tube radios so often donated to institutions and used for training purposes.

3. The mixing and timing of different kinds of course work is also important. Many clients need remedial education in the "3 R's." If possible, this can be integrated in the training program where appropriate, or dealt with concurrently by a specialist.

4. Incentives should be built into the learning process itself, since the ultimate incentive, gainful employment, may appear too distant and unreal to the client. Incentives offered in the past to trainees have been program insignias, proficiency certificates, class trophies, and graduation exercises, in addition to money. The nature of the incentive, of course, should be selected according to the specific client and to the unique situation in the facility.

The Termination of Services

The termination of rehabilitation services should be a positive experience for the public offender client and, hopefully, represent a success in his very probable long list of failures. For this reason, timing becomes very important in this phase of the rehabilitation process. Successful rehabilitation of the public offenders generally requires a considerably longer period of time than rehabilitation agencies and facilities are used to affording. The increased time may not necessarily be in terms of a single period in a facility, but rather in terms of a lengthy follow-up and support period after leaving a facility program. A client should not be expected to leave the program and become an overnight success in the community. But rather, once again, problems can be expected to crop up and the facility should keep its doors open for as long as is necessary. Some overdependency will be observed in clients from time to time but this will become a real problem in relatively few cases. A reasonable amount of dependency can be expected in a good number of clients. This is a necessary part of the rehabilitation process and has been fostered by the facility program. Most generally, with the proper timing and supportive counseling, this dependency will be dissolved.

Follow-up services should be an integral part of the total program of any facility serving public offender clients. It is a very important but often neglected phase in the rehabilitation process. Not only will a good follow-up program add needed support to the client, it will also allow the facility a means for the evaluation of its efforts.

REFERENCES

Diagnostic and Statistical Manual of Mental Disorders, 2d ed. American Psychiatric Association, 1968.

Glasser, D.: *The Effectiveness of a Prison and Parole System.* New York, Bobbs-Merrill, 1964.

Hardy, R. E. and Cull, J. G.: *Introduction to Correctional Rehabilitation.* Springfield, Charles C Thomas, 1973.

Stratten, J.: Correctional workers: Counseling con men? *Federal Probation,* 37:3, 1973.

CHAPTER 7

VOCATIONAL REHABILITATION OF THE OLDER AMERICAN IN REHABILITATION FACILITIES

ROLAND BAXT and ALFRED P. MILLER

I N DISCUSSING the best way to proceed with the development of a chapter on vocational rehabilitation of the older American in the rehabilitation facility, the authors were deeply concerned with creating a relevant resource for practitioners and administrators who are currently working with handicapped elderly and aged and for those who will be or should be working with elderly and aged handicapped individuals.

It was decided to divide the chapter into three sections:

Section I deals with the background of vocational rehabilitation services for the older American, the experiences of the Federation Employment and Guidance Service which helped to pioneer some of these services, and pertinent statistics demonstrating the scope of the problem as well as what has been accomplished to date.

In *Section II* the authors have decided to present a format of questions and answers. These questions were gathered at a series of meetings the authors held with practitioners and administrators working with the vocational rehabilitation needs of the aged, as well as with practitioners working with other disability groups. It is hoped that by using this format, practitioners will feel part of a seminar-type approach rather than a lecture approach to the problems encountered, expectations, and actual experience obtained over many years of working with the vocational rehabilitation of the elderly and aged. The questions and answers concern themselves with the specific characteristics of this population as differentiated from other disabled populations, including physical plant and equipment, the personality

119

characteristics of the population, unique problems of the aged and their effects on practitioners and the rehabilitation process, the type of vocational rehabilitation environment felt to be best suited for working with the aged, job placement problems, skills training problems, funding, funding sources, staffing patterns, cooperating agencies and their attitudes toward the elderly and aged in both public and private agencies, counselor attitudes toward the aged, types of contract work for workshops, effect on cost of production of an aged population *vis-à-vis* a younger population, programmatic approaches and attitudes toward the aged, including employer attitudes toward the aged and community attitudes, and motivation factors and behavioral characteristics of the aged as contrasted to other groups.

Since all pertinent areas could not be covered in a single section of a single chapter, the authors feel that this format might also encourage students and those interested in the vocational rehabilitation of the aged who find themselves with questions not discussed in the chapter to write to the authors or to the Federation Employment and Guidance Service for a further discussion of those questions.

Section III is a summary section discussing the need for advocacy, where we are now, and where do we go from here in rehabilitation services for the elderly and aged. This section describes the FEGS model of a vocational rehabilitation service delivery system.

Background of Services for the Older American

In the United States the social welfare system developed under government and voluntary auspices was designed to serve a particular group and to meet a particular need at a particular time. Areas of need, which in some other countries are regarded as proper concern of social policy, are in our country regarded as a prerogative of the individual.

Our support of national welfare programs has been somewhat halting. Yet, we move forward, griping a little as we go along. In the past twenty years ideas which seemed radical are currently supported by many government committees and groups with impeccable credentials, e.g. Medicare and Vocational Rehabilitation for the older American.

The following are some excerpts from a recent report on aging prepared by the United Nations: "In another twenty years, there will be 585 million people sixty years of age and over. This will represent about 16 percent of the population in the developed countries." The report concludes that one of the most crucial social policy questions for the remainder of the twentieth century is the aging. The report (Isn't This Much of What Vocational Rehabilitation Is All About?) urges programs be devised not only on a crisis basis, but also for preventive and development purposes. The report asserts the right of all older persons to services and facilities directed at helping them participate and contribute to society. The report stresses helping the aged remain in their own homes as long as possible as an alternative to institutionalization. One of the best models of this for the severely disabled aged is the long-term vocational rehabilitation facility for service on the premises and in the home.

Basic to the concept underlying a vocational rehabilitation program for older disabled persons is a recognition of the rights of people in our system, regardless of age, to try to meet their legitimate needs through socially accepted channels that are provided all citizens. Past and current vocational rehabilitation legislation, federal and state, does not specify an upper age limit. It is important to note that the 1973 federal vocational rehabilitation legislation, perhaps for the first time, identifies the aged for special study as to their service needs. Also of great significance is the Administration on Aging legislative mandate which requires special treatment to the physically and mentally handicapped aged.

The feasibility of vocational rehabilitation for the aged has been demonstrated again and again. The prototype which was set up in the VRA days, based on Federation Employment and Guidance Service (FEGS) research and demonstration on feasibility of vocational rehabilitation for persons disabled and sixty years of age and over, was duplicated in at least eleven states and the Virgin Islands, with a 75 percent or more rehabilitation success.

The U. S. Department of Health, Education and Welfare-Social and Rehabilitation Service-Rehabilitation Services Administration reported that in the 1972 year 326,138 individuals were rehabilitated. More than 30 percent were forty-five years of age and over, including 6.5 percent that were sixty-five years of age and over. Reports from the same source also state "the mean costs for case service *declines* with increasing age for those who are rehabilitated."

At the 1971 White House Conference on Aging, some three thousand delegates, representing some fifty million people, urged those who deliver vocational rehabilitation services to serve more older eligible applicants, at least those who are motivated and want to achieve partial or full-time support and have all the other benefits which result from rehabilitation services.

The authors of this chapter and the agency with which they are affiliated have been advocates for many years for vocational rehabilitation services for the aged. We will try in what we hope will be an effective format to raise and answer the pertinent questions which concern practitioners, administrators, and sponsors.

Basic Aspects of Older American Rehabilitation

Question

What are some of the myths held by the general public and even some practitioners regarding the abilities and capabilities of the handicapped elderly and aged?

Answer

It is common for the general public and even some practitioners to hold preconceived beliefs or myths about various handicapped populations; the cerebral palsied cannot work on assembly items in a workshop or the mentally retarded can only do the most menial tasks. However, in the case of the elderly and aged handicapped there is an extra dimension. The general public and some practitioners tend to relate in some way the elderly and aged handicapped with their parent or grandparent, particularly when they have arrived at an advanced age. Many of them think in terms of protectiveness—of protecting grandpa or grandma from doing anything that exerts energy, in attempting to make all decisions for grandpa or grandma, in relating to nursing homes and institutionalization as the place for the advanced aged handicapped individual. Therefore, everyone tends to be an expert in knowing what the elderly and aged handicapped can and cannot do. At least in the areas of other disability groups one might question the fact that they have not worked with such groups or have not had direct contact with such groups as raising at least a doubt as to what the limitations of members of such a disability group are. Some of the myths that are widely held about the elderly and aged handicapped in a vocational rehabilitation program are as follows: they do not want to work; they worked hard enough all their lives, and they should have a recreation program, but not necessarily a vocational rehabilitation program; their mental processes have slowed down to a point where skills training cannot be absorbed properly; with limited resources, why should we spend money training an individual fifty, sixty or sixty-five years old in a skill where he can work in that occupation for another five or ten years; the elderly and aged are not interested in job advancement or are not willing or able to travel; they have more accidents than younger people; they miss more days of work due to illness; they can never be on time for work. We could go on and list many more beliefs held by the general public and some practitioners, but the fact is that the elderly and aged have the same limitations and the same desires and the same goals in life as other age groups. Generalizations are as fallacious of an elderly and aged population as they are of the younger generation—disabled and non-disabled. An elderly aged and handicapped individual must be helped vocationally as an individual.

Question

What are some of the unique problems of the handicapped elderly and aged, and what effect do these problems have on the practitioner and on the rehabilitation process itself?

Answer

Some problems are unique to the handicapped elderly and aged, in addition to those problems related to the specific disability. One of the major problems confronting the practitioner and the rehabilitation process itself is that on the whole, the aged population is not an outspoken group until they get to know the particular counselor or feel comfortable in the rehabilitation facility. They are usually fearful of losing some sort of limited income, such as Social Security, a pension or some other income which relates to the amount of money they are able to earn. In many cases, they dislike a direct confrontation with the problem, and therefore skirt around the issue making up many excuses for not wanting to do something or for not accepting a certain type of work adjustment or training because they are fearful of either losing some income or of the effect such training might have on their family situation. For example, they may be obligated to babysit for a grandchild, and, while the counselor may very well be able to talk to the son or daughter about making other arrangements that would enable the client to take part in the training program, the counselor must be experienced in working with the geriatric population in ferreting out the real reason why the client may be hesitant to take part in a program.

While it is true that this can be said to some degree about other disabled populations and that this is part of the normal technique of counseling, it is our feeling, based on our experience and in talking to other practitioners serving the geriatric population, that this kind of problem is more prevalent among the geriatric population.

Another problem that is often encountered is that many of the clients in the geriatric population have worked at one trade all of their lives and are hesitant and frightened about learning a new skill or technique or a different kind of job. They require a great deal of sympathetic understanding and a great deal of explanation about the type of training and the type of rehabilitation program being recommended to them. This touches a bit on the answer to our next question.

Question

What type of counselor would you say is better suited to working with an elderly and aged population? Does an elderly or younger counselor relate better to an elderly and aged population?

Answer

This is a difficult question that has been discussed regarding all types of disability groups. Is an ex-drug addict better able to deal with an ex-drug abuse population? Is an ex-alcoholic better able to deal with an ex-alcoholic population? Let us make it clear at the beginning that it is our belief that a good counselor, well prepared and well trained, can work with any disability population. However, we should note that we have found that in the early stages of developing a rapport with an elderly or aged handicapped individual, the elderly person may be more receptive to a chronologically older person and may be more open in the discussion of his problems. However, a younger person can overcome this initial difficulty by bringing to the counseling process a higher degree of maturity and some training in dealing with the geriatric population.

Question

What are the most common questions asked by the handicapped elderly or aged person of the counselor in a rehabilitation center or workshop?

Answer

Since we do not wish to create our own myths about the elderly and aged, we must, in responding to this question, state that the elderly and aged handicapped person, being an individual, can ask any question as can anyone else. However, generally speaking, questions that seem to be asked over and over again by a geriatric population in a rehabilitation center or workshop generally revolve around areas of economics, safety, and job security. They are concerned, as mentioned previously, with the possible loss of their pensions or social security benefits. They are concerned about how much they can earn on a job, and the neighborhood in which they will have to work. In many cases they are concerned about whether they would be accepted by the population with whom they would be working, and how long they can expect to keep a job when they can get one. There is a great deal of feeling of insecurity that they will be let go when a younger person comes along. How much will they earn while they are in a training program, and how long will the training program last?

In most cases, this population is truly one of rehabilitation and not of re-habilitation. These are people who have worked all of their lives and believe in the work ethic. In many cases they consider it degrading and demoralizing to earn a relatively small amount of money, whether it be a training stipend or a piece-work rate on subcontract work in a workshop. A man who has been a cutter in the garment industry or a shoemaker or a cabinet maker and can no longer do this type of work but who may have the ability and capability of learning to do a skilled job in another area resents bitterly being pushed into a messenger job, primarily because of his advanced age and disability. He may sense or imagine in the counselor a feeling that he or she, in some way, is less than what he or she was, and as such may become defensive and arbitrarily refuse anything that the counselor may suggest. It is important that the counselor, in recognizing this, make an effort to explore in detail the client's past vocational history and current vocational desires in attempting to plan a vocational rehabilitation program with the client.

Question

Are there barriers to employment that are unique to the elderly and aged?

Answer

There are barriers to employment that can be considered unique to the elderly and aged, especially since we are a youth-oriented society. Employer receptivity is geared to the young. In addition, there are some very real economic barriers such as a limitation due to Social Security and pension benefits as to how much the client can earn. There is a great deal of hesitancy among the elderly and aged to give up some part of Social Security and pension benefits which they feel they have worked all their lives to earn. Transportation, while a barrier to all disability groups, is certainly a severe barrier to the elderly and aged, especially when combined in large urban areas with the problems of safety and the fact that the elderly and aged are often singled out as targets for mugging and robbery. Sometimes the problem is social with the family; a son or daughter can make the parent feel that he or she is responsible for babysitting with a grandchild, or they may feel that any work is too difficult for mom or pop at age sixty-five or more, without taking into regard the feelings or the needs of mom or pop.

Question

Are there special skills or education necessary for rehabilitation counselors who wish to work with the geriatric population?

Answer

The authors believe that there should certainly be some added emphasis in the rehabilitation counseling education programs on working with the geriatric disabled population. In addition, we believe that any exposure to a geriatric population by way of an internship practicum or fellowship would enable the graduate student and future practitioners to become more aware of the behavioral characteristics of the geriatric population. This would enable the future practitioners to obtain a firsthand knowledge of Social Security and pension limitations and their effect on this population, as well as to become familiar with the physical characteristics and family and social relationships. These include the fear of being institutionalized or being sent to a nursing home, the fear of children deserting them or not giving them the respect to which they feel they are entitled, and the fear that society is changing all around them at such a rapid pace that they are strangers in their own environment. The changing social mores of the younger population in relationship to the elderly and aged and the apparent breakdown of the family structure are all elements which the rehabilitation counselor and future practitioner should at least become aware of in order to successfully work with a geriatric population in a vocational rehabilitation setting.

Question

Is the cost per client or the cost per rehabilitation higher for older people than it is for younger people with the same disability?

Answer

Research into the cost per rehabilitation for an elderly population as related to that of the cost for the younger tends to show that the mean costs decline with increasing age. Costs of case service as reported by the Rehabilitation Services Administration bear this out in regard to case service. This could be due partially to the fact that the aged are not being given sufficient skills, training opportunities, or long-term opportunities that are given to some younger population, but it also indicates that the costs are not higher for an elderly person than for a younger person. However, the authors have found that in their own agency's experience, as well as in talking with other administrators and practitioners who have worked with a geriatric population, that a large number of disabled geriatric clients require long-term care or long-term sheltered workshop programs. In some states, this is considered part of the rehabilitation program, and a fee for services is paid by the state's vocational rehabilitation service to the agencies providing long-term services. But, in most states, there is no fee for service, and many of the elderly and aged are not given the opportunity to be part of a long-term workshop program. Although this would increase the cost of maintaining such an individual in a long-term vocational rehabilitation program, it would fill one of the greatest unmet needs in vocational rehabilitation services for the disabled elderly and aged, a larger percentage of whom require long-term services than a younger group with the same disability.

Question

What are the special requirements for physical plant—that is, what type of rehabilitation facility is necessary in order to serve a disabled geriatric population?

Answer

To the best of our knowledge and experience, there are no special requirements for physical plant or type of rehabilitation facility which are specifically different in serving a geriatric disability population than in serving a similarly disabled younger group.

It depends primarily on the type of disability in deciding what types of jigs or special machinery or equipment or aisles or fire alarm systems or safety precautions are necessary in a rehabilitation facility. The location of the facility, however, particularly in larger cities, could be of primary importance. Large cities which are divided into many neighborhoods, sometimes as in New York numbering in the hundreds, create for those who have resided in those neighborhoods for thirty, forty, fifty or more years a certain lifestyle, a certain rigidity and a certain dislike for change in the elderly and aged that can affect their vocational rehabilitation program as well as their eventual job placement. They seem to adapt better to a vocational rehabilitation facility or place of employment located in their own neighborhood than they do when they have to travel to a central office, rehabilitation facility, or employer. This is not as true of the younger population which is more adaptable and which has not accepted the same kind of rigid lifestyle.

The size of the facility does not seem to have any special significance. However, the population mix within the facility does. It has been our experience that in a geriatric vocational rehabilitation facility serving all disability groups, the elderly and aged population play a significant role in serving as a model of stability to a younger population, particularly one with behavior problems that may act out frequently. However, having a younger behavioral problem population in the same facility seems to adversely affect the vocational rehabilitation program of the elderly and aged population. It causes disruption in their day-to-day program. It could create fear and anxiety in the older population, and could cause early dropout of the elderly and aged clients from the program.

Question

Is there a greater problem of rigidity as well as resistance on the part of the elderly person to counselor's suggestions than on the part of the younger person, and is there a difference between an elderly group of forty-five to sixty-five as opposed to an aged group of sixty-five and over?

Answer

We touched on this area in an earlier question. There is a greater resistance and problem of rigidity on the part of an older person to a counselor's recommendation and suggestions, but to a great extent, this may be due primarily to the particular characteristic of the older disabled population not to confront a problem head on. By so doing, his reaction to a counselor's suggestion may appear to be rigid where in effect it is his way of asking for help or a solution to a problem, but the counselor must ferret out the problem with great skill. The counselor must have a great deal of knowledge of the labor market and of various occupations. He must have an understanding of the type of work the client has done all of his life. He must understand the pride that a skilled tradesman or craftsman has taken in the work he has done previously. He must understand the great need for dignity and respect that the elderly and aged require. He must be extra careful not to give the impression that he is talking down to them, especially if the counselor is a younger counselor. The counselor must not fight the apparent rigidity or responses on the part of the older client, but must attempt to find out what the cause of such resistance is.

There is a definite difference between an elderly group—forty-five to sixty-five—and an aged group of sixty-five and over in the degree of resistance or rigidity that is apparent. There are other differences between these two groups. The younger group tends to be in a rehabilitation program primarily due to some accident or illness which has necessitated their requiring vocational rehabilitation services. This manifests itself in an abrupt change that this group now faces, whereas the elderly group has usually had more time to adjust to the causes requiring vocational rehabilitation services. The techniques in dealing with these two groups of population obviously differ.

Question

Are there different staffing patterns necessary for rehabilitation facilities serving the elderly and aged?

Answer

There are basic staffing patterns that are necessary for rehabilitation facilities serving the elderly and aged. They tend to require less career counseling and more intensive diagnostic vocational evaluation. It is not so much that they are confused vocationally, but that they require a more intensive work evaluation and medical evaluation in order to determine what their abilities and capabilities are. Thus, there would be a greater need for evaluators and evaluation systems, such as the Tower, the Philadelphia JVS system, the Singer Graflex or the like, plus a greater need for an on or off premises actual work evaluation program. We will discuss this type of programming in the summary section of this chapter.

Question

How does one establish linkages between a public agency and a private agency in order to expand and improve services to a geriatric population?

Answer

The authors believe strongly that an integral part of counseling is a belief on the part of the practitioner that his or her clients are entitled to all of the services necessary in order to accomplish a successful vocational rehabilitation. As such, the counselor, whether working for the public agency or the private agency, becomes an advocate for the clients he serves.

One of the necessary ways of improving services for any population, but especially for a disabled geriatric population, is to establish better linkages between the public agency and the private agency. This is a multiple level function. Linkages should be established from administrator to administrator in terms of program funding and in terms of making certain that the elderly and aged get their fair share of the funding available. But, it is also a counselor to counselor linkage, sharing information as to the progress of programming for an elderly and aged population, as to the needs required, as to the capability and potential of a population being served, and in order to break down any myths being held by practitioners both in the public and private agency and by the public. It is also important for the practitioner and administrator and members of the Board to carry this linkage to their professional associations and to obtain from the professional associations a commitment toward increasing and enriching vocational rehabilitation services for the elderly and aged. It is important to get community support for such programs and to educate the public as to the needs and abilities and desires of the disabled geriatric population vis-à-vis vocational rehabilitation services.

Question

What are some of the motivation factors and behavior characteristics of the aged in contrast to the younger disabled groups?

Answer

This is another area in which we must generalize to make our point. However, we must also note once again that among any group of individuals, there are differences to the general rule. Basically, the elderly and aged disabled client is a well motivated individual, vocationally speaking. As mentioned previously, he believes in the work ethic. He has worked most of his active life; he does not have to be sold on the concept of work. Generally speaking, he does not present behavioral problems while he is in work adjustment or skills training programs, but he may be suffering from depression, from a sense of failure, from a belief that he has wasted many of his years, from a feeling of inadequacy, from a sense of hopelessness that his life as a productive member of society is nearing an end, from a fear of an uncertain and unknown future, from family problems, and from a youth-oriented system.

These create certain behavior characteristics which are in marked contrast to many of the younger disabled groups. These can manifest themselves in evasiveness, abruptness, apparent rigidity, a certain resentfulness, an unwillingness to accept advice from a counselor, a feeling that certain work in a workshop might be too demeaning for him or her, and a constant feeling that he is being discriminated against, especially in a workshop with a mixed population of younger and older disabled groups. For example, if he sees a younger client working faster and producing more, he may feel tempted to ask: "Why are you giving him better work then you are giving me?," or "Why did so and so make more money last week?," or "Why was client *B* sent out on a job instead of me?" This is not a behavior characteristic representing true anger or general griping, but is a reflection more of a feeling of inadequacy and fear on the part of the older person. It must be met with a sympathetic understanding on the part of the counselor if he is to achieve a working rapport with his client.

Question

Does it make sense to offer skills training programs with limited funding to the handicapped elderly and aged when they have so few years left in which to work in the labor market?

Answer

This is a question which the authors have repeatedly been asked. This is really a policy decision that must be made by the government. We can only give our viewpoint as to whether or not it makes sense to offer skills training programs while funding is limited to a handicapped elderly and aged population rather than reserving it for a younger disabled and disadvantaged population.

We have demonstrated, as have many others, that a man or woman aged sixty or sixty-five or older can be trained in a school, can be placed in a job in industry, and can work successfully for another five, ten or even fifteen years. It is our strong belief that an individual, disabled or non-disabled, who has the motivation and desire to learn and improve himself should be given every opportunity to do so. Who is to deny an individual this opportunity because he only has ten or fifteen years of a working life remaining? We believe that funding should be shared equally among all those who need it, without special funding being reserved for any one disability group or age group. If there is not enough, it is up to the practitioners in the field who serve as advocates to see that more is made available rather than to deny services that have been demonstrated to improve the lifestyle of an individual and to improve his economic status.

Question

Can the elderly and aged absorb skills training, new techniques and knowledge rapidly enough to hope for a successful job placement and vocational rehabilitation in a competitive labor market?

Answer

As we have touched on in answering the previous question, we have been convinced over the years, observing various research, demonstration and service programs both in our own agency and in other agencies, that the elderly and aged handicapped client has the motivation and the ability to absorb skills training in areas which employ new technology and which he may not have come in contact with before. It may take him a little longer to master these techniques than a younger population with a similar disability, but he can successfully complete a skills training program and apply these skills after job placement in the competitive labor market.

In many cases, employers have reported to us that they lose less days with an older and aged population who are not only motivated to do the work but who are grateful at having obtained the training and the job, and bring to the job a level of maturity which in the long run probably gives the employer the same if not greater production than he obtains from his younger employees.

Question

Do you believe that we should have separate facilities for the handicapped elderly and aged during the rehabilitation process?

Answer

In responding to an earlier question, we had noted that while we believe that the elderly and aged present a good training and work model to a younger and more diversified disabled population in a generic workshop or facility, we have also seen evidence that the effect of some of these younger populations with behavior problems can have on the elderly and aged, increasing within them a feeling of anxiety, fear, and sometimes causing early dropout from the program among the elderly and aged clients. This can be somewhat controlled by more intensive counseling on the part of both the younger and older populations.

The decision as to whether to have separate facilities is one that depends upon the resources available, the objectives of the rehabilitation agency, and the needs of the community. It is our belief that if it is possible to have a separate facility for the elderly and aged, they would probably be more comfortable, but we must question whether they would be receiving adequate training for working in a non-sheltered environment where they are going to be with all age groups, all ethnic groups and the population in general. We would therefore sum up our position as saying that while we would recommend separate facilities for long-term or extended workshop clients who are elderly and aged, we would not recommend it for those in a transitional workshop who are in evaluation, work adjustment or skills training programs, and for whom the objective is employment in competitive industry.

Question

Are the elderly and aged aware of vocational rehabilitation programs? Is it more necessary to establish reach-out programs for this population than it is for a younger population?

Answer

Experience has demonstrated to us that the disability group most unaware of vocational rehabilitation programs and of vocational rehabilitation services available to them are the elderly and aged disabled. Most of these people grew up at a time when the programs available today and the government funding available today for such programs were not available. Many of them have the feeling of relating all government sponsored programs to welfare programs, and as economically deprived as many of them may be, a large number of them shun welfare as a matter of pride and dignity.

Therefore, it is necessary to have an extensive reach-out and education program to explain the services that are available to them, to explain their right to such services, to differentiate the multitude of services in different areas that may be available in a community, and to attempt to help the disabled elderly and aged to select the kind of service he requires and then to show him how he can obtain such services. Sometimes, it is necessary for the vocational rehabilitation facility itself to provide outstationing of staff on a temporary basis to housing projects, community centers, Y's, and medical centers in order to help to actually register those who need vocational rehabilitation services in an attempt to cut through some of the red tape of the intake and eligibility process. After all, six months' or a year's delay in obtaining service for a man or woman who is sixty-five or seventy is certainly a luxury they cannot afford.

While reach-out is necessary for disabled populations of all ages, there are many more government sponsored reach-out programs designed to reach the younger population than there are for the elderly and aged. Hence, the rehabilitation facility must feel that it must act once again as an advocate for the elderly and aged handicapped in what is more and more a youth-oriented system.

Question

Are there differences between vocational rehabilitation planning for handicapped elderly and aged who have worked all their lives in a professional or clerical capacity and those who have worked in blue-collar or factory jobs, between male and female, between native-born and foreign-born, and between rural and urban elderly and aged, in terms of planning a vocational rehabilitation program?

Answer

There are differences among individuals who may be the same age and have the same disability, were born and brought up in the same neighborhood, and have worked in the same occupation all of their lives. Considering this, one can begin to see that there can be vast differences between elderly and aged disabled who have worked in a professional or clerical capacity and those who have worked in blue-collar or factory jobs, between native-born and foreign-born, between rural and urban, and between male and female. Vocational rehabilitation programs must, therefore, be geared so that they are flexible enough and offer enough of a variety of rehabilitation and training opportunities to meet the needs of these different groups of elderly and aged disabled. They cannot and should not be fitted into one mold labelled "rehabilitation services for the elderly and disabled." A woman who has worked at clerical work all her life may find it very demeaning to be placed at a work bench in a workshop assembling fountain pens every day. A man who has worked on a farm all his life may find it extremely difficult to work in a factory, and vice versa.

This was one of the major reasons why the authors and FEGS have created a vocational rehabilitation program which is both flexible and open ended, which offers a variety of evaluation, work adjustment and skills training opportunities which can be tailored to the individual needs of an individual elderly and aged disabled client. This model is described in Section III, or the summary section of this chapter.

Summary

There are many models for a vocational rehabilitation program serving the elderly and aged as well as other disability groups. Although we have touched upon many of the areas of service offered to the aged, we would like to present in the summary section one model for a programmatic approach of a service delivery system that we are using at the Federation Employment and Guidance Service in our vocational rehabilitation program for the elderly and aged. We must note here that this model is flexible and subject to changes. It is possible for someone to extract from it sections or parts that one might use in establishing their own vocational rehabilitation service for the elderly and aged while discarding other sections. Although this model has been developed for a very large agency, the basic approach could be utilized in small and medium sized agencies. We have designed our program to be geographically decentralized in order to bring services closer to where individuals requiring such service reside. We felt that this was necessary because of the nature and vastness of New York City. The same programmatic approach can be developed for a rehabilitation facility located in a single structure in a moderate sized community.

FEGS offers a broad range of vocational rehabilitation services for the aged as well as for other disability groups. These services allow the FEGS' staff to individualize the rehabilitation program to help meet the vocational need of each client. Our programmatic approach resembles a career ladder toward vocational rehabilitation. An outline of the structure is as follows.

Diagnostic Vocational Evaluation

Clients enter a diagnostic vocational work sample evaluation as a result of which a determination is made as to the type of program which best suits the client rather that the type of program for which the client is best suited. By this we mean that we have made every effort to individualize the programs to meet the individualized need of the clients. The evaluation team may suggest any one of the following programs for the client:

1. If the primary need is for work adjustment in a sheltered environment in order to create the basis necessary for any successful vocational rehabilitation, the client may be referred to the vocational rehabilitation facility in the Bronx, Brooklyn, Queens or Manhattan which most closely approximates the area they reside in for a period of personal adjustment or work adjustment training, during which he works on real subcontract work and is paid for the work he performs based on the prevailing wage in industry. During this time, he is given intensive supportive counseling and intensive supervision.

2. If the primary need is for work adjustment in a semi-sheltered or less sheltered environment with the secondary need of skills training, the client is placed in an aides' station. This is usually located in a nonprofit institution, such as a hospital, home for the aged, social agency, school or government agency, an aides' station which has been selected for him based on the evaluation. For example, the evaluation team has projected the possibility of gardening. However, before the client can really learn gardening or be placed on a job in competitive industry, he may have a far greater immediate need of work adjustment. He might be placed as a gardener's aide in a hospital. Aides' stations range from maintenance aide to X-ray technician aide and library aide.

3. Where the individual's primary immediate need is skills training with a secondary need of work adjustment, a determination is made as to whether this need can best be met in a sheltered or non-sheltered environment. If a sheltered environment is selected for the client, he would be referred to one of the agency's institutional vocational skills training programs nearest his residence. This range includes porter, maintenance, typing, switchboard, junior bookkeeping, typewriter repair and business machine repair, jewelry production and repair, basic electric, machine shop, and other

occupational training areas. The training is given on the premises under close supervision with intensive supportive counseling. If the semi-sheltered or unsheltered skills training operation is selected, the agency conducts an intensive job station in industry program. This is where training is conducted on the employer's own premises under a formal OJT with a regular curriculum and time-frame established for the training. The job station's coordinating team has created a job bank of job station slots which range across the occupational spectrum. These include gem polisher, picture framemaker, auto mechanic, gemsetter, business machine repairman, dental assistant, and a variety of other occupations. The individual may be referred upon completion of evaluation to one of these job stations as well as in the job station's bank. It may be necessary for the job station's coordinator to seek out a job station not already in the bank in accordance with the request by the evaluation team for an individual client.

4. For those individuals who cannot meet the demands for employment in the private sector, the agency conducts a long-term care program of long-term sheltered employment in its facilities. The long-term program consists of: a) production subcontract work for which clients are paid a piece-work rate; b) long-term skills training contract program where clients work on contracts in the area for which they have been trained, receiving a piece-work rate for work performed, and c) government contract programs of a service and/or production component (Wagner-O'Day), in which clients are paid the prevailing wage rate in industry (usually around $2.00 per hour). Since FEGS firmly believes that this is not just a long-term employment program but a long-term rehabilitation program, all clients in long-term status are reevaluated, medically and vocationally, every three months to determine their availability for a job in competitive industry. Many are placed on jobs in the private sector after three, five or eight years in long-term status.

The following is a more detailed description of what we do during the evaluation phase of the client's program.

All clients enter diagnostic work sample evaluation. During this phase of their program, clients are evaluated in order to determine:

1. The barriers to employment which prevent this particular client from obtaining suitable employment at this particular time. This might involve the basics of work adjustment, such as ability to accept supervision, peer relationships, punctuality, work tolerance, and self-image as a worker, or it may involve lack of saleable skills of any kind, or it may involve the need for basic remediation in reading, arithmetic, English as a Second Language, high school equivalency preparation, or it may involve a period of pre-employment work adjustment.

2. A projection as to the client's abilities and capabilities and selection of career training is accomplished through:
   a. Work samples
   b. Psychological testing
   c. Observation by the evaluator of the client in the work situation
   d. The client's workshop performance
   e. Counseling interviews
   f. Supervisor and foreman observations and reports
   g. Review of medical, psycho-social and vocational information

An enlarged and enriched program of work samples is used as an integral part of the evaluation. This approach helps us to understand a client's vocational potential and needs more fully. These work samples have been correlated to occupational aptitude patterns, and were originally developed by our sister agency, the Philadelphia Jewish Employment and Vocational Service, and modified by FEGS.

The following work samples are used by us in the evaluation process:

1. Proofreading
2. Collating of Leather Sample
3. Use of Adding Machine
4. Sign Making
5. Rubber Stamping

6. Lock Assembly
7. Nut Boxing
8. Tile Sorting
9. Coupling Operation
10. Belt Assembly
11. Foot Press Operation
12. Bindery Operation
13. Payroll Computation
14. Ladder Assembly
15. Washer Threading
16. Nail and Screw Sorting
17. Pipefitter Operation
18. Swatch Cutting
19. Telephone Assembly
20. Bell Assembly
21. Soldering Operation
22. Filing—Numerically & Alphabetically
23. Typing
24. Weighing Items & Computation of Postage
25. Zoning Postage
26. Nut, Bolt and Washer Assembly

Additional work samples are available, and are used selectively as needed. The work sample approach is reality-oriented and this is its major virtue. It is a close simulation of actual work demands and since it is administered in a reasonably controlled industrial setting, it is an unparalleled opportunity to observe basic employment behavior. The tasks are simulated job duties and not a formal test situation, and it is assumed that the individual, being less defensive, is more prone to assert his capabilities and thus will reveal his potential cognitive, conative and affective self-pattern. By observing the performance of an individual undergoing work sample evaluation, the evaluator and vocational counselors increase their scope of information. This helps to generate more valid hypotheses about the client's employability because the evaluator-counselor derives richer insights than would be possible from a standard battery of psychometric tests. The procedure does not attempt to pinpoint specific occupational objectives, but is designed to assist in the determination of one's ability for fields of work or job families. They are not selection instruments and should not be used as such. However, they are rather concrete situations that examine the degree to which the individual can adapt and perform according to a set of prescribed demands.

The work samples being used by the Federation Employment and Guidance Service at the present time are validated and normed in the same manner as standard psychometric tests. This norming and validation allow their use in a precise and scientific manner, making resulting judgments concerning client performance and potential much more accurate and meaningful.

Based on our initial observations, we have come to a tentative finding that work samples may cut down on the rate of dropout for clients who go through this process as their first point of contact.

Work Adjustment and Skills Training

On the basis of the results and findings of the vocational evaluation, the client will enter one of the following:

1. Sheltered work adjustment at an FEGS Vocational Rehabilitation Center.
2. Aides' station work adjustment both on and off the FEGS premises, including nonprofit and government agencies.
3. Institutional skills training in a sheltered environment at an FEGS Skills Training Center in the following skills training areas: mailroom, messenger, reproduction machine operator, switchboard operator, clerk-typist, file clerk, junior bookkeeping, bookkeeping, business machine repair, jewelry production and repair, basic electric, and machine shop.
4. Skills training off premises at job sites (job stations in industry) set up as a formal OJT on the employer's premises with full supportive counseling.
5. Long-term sheltered workshop program.
6. Long-term skills training program.
7. Long-term government contract program (Wagner O'Day).

During this phase of the client's program, he will be provided with continuing remediation services in arithmetic, reading skills as well as English as a second language, and if appropriate, high school equivalency preparation and business math, as needed. Classes are conducted by experienced and qualified teachers. Throughout the client's entire program, he will be afforded constant vocational counseling on a periodic and as needed basis. In addition, referrals are made to other agencies in the community network for other identified non-vocational services.

Job Placement

At any time commencing with the referral of the client to FEGS by the referring agency, the client will initially be considered for placement. If referral is made by the FEGS Intake Unit to the FEGS Vocational Rehabilitation Program, he need not necessarily complete the FEGS rehabilitation program, or for that matter, enter the vocational rehabilitation program after completion of the initial stage of diagnostic work sample evaluation. As soon as the client is deemed ready for placement, he is placed on a job. Sometimes this will be an entry level job with supportive and upgrading services rendered after the initial placement.

The length of time a client is scheduled to be in a particular phase of his rehabilitation program is flexible. The objective is to secure a proper placement for each client at the earliest possible time, although taking care not to make a premature placement before the client has acquired the appropriate skills and work behavior. It is also not necessary for the client to enter each phase of the program successively. It is possible to go directly from evaluation into a job station or job placement without ever entering a formal work adjustment phase. In other words, the program, although tightly structured, offers the opportunity for individual planning around the needs of each individual client.

All clients are offered *follow-along services* commencing with the referral to possible job openings. In some cases, the placement counselor may personally accompany the client to the job interview. In other cases, the employer will be called at predetermined phases of the client's work adjustment after placement, such as the first payday, in an attempt to encourage the employer to be patient and to continue the client's employment, or the week prior to a client's being allowed to join the union at the end of his probationary period. The intervention of the placement counselor at these given points has proven to be effective. Problems may be discussed at that time, and these can then be brought to the attention of the client in an effort to resolving them and to eliminate a possible emerging barrier to continued employment. Should the client fail to make a positive adjustment after placement, he may return to one of the agency's long-term programs, and the counseling, adjustment and placement process (where indicated) repeated.

We believe that a comprehensive structured yet flexible vocational adjustment program such as this model enhances greatly the probability of a successful vocational rehabilitation.

Although we have seen in Section II that there are a great many unique problems presented by a handicapped elderly and aged population in the vocational rehabilitation process, we have also seen that many of the problems are not so vastly different between a handicapped elderly and a handicapped younger individual. We have also seen, however, that the myths built around the vocational rehabilitation of the elderly and aged do abound and that on the part of the community, the public and private agencies, the counselors and practitioners, a great deal more of specialized preparation for the professional planning to work in the vocational rehabilitation of the elderly and aged is required.

Working with any disability group in the vocational rehabilitation field carries with it the obligation on the part of the practitioner and the administrator to carry forth a program of education of the public and advocacy for that population in order to obtain their fair share of services and funding. A constant seeking of new methods and new programmatic approaches which can help to decrease the time and funds necessary to achieve a successful vocational rehabilitation is needed. It is also their obligation to prepare the individual for the highest level of employment he is capable of achieving, and to follow that

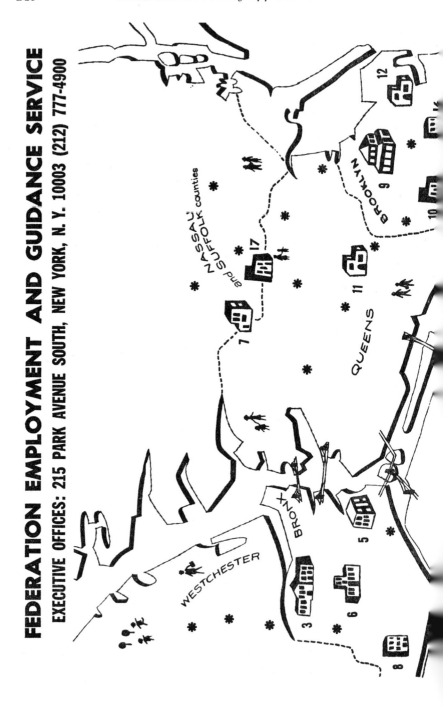

FEDERATION EMPLOYMENT AND GUIDANCE SERVICE

EXECUTIVE OFFICES: 215 PARK AVENUE SOUTH, NEW YORK, N. Y. 10003 (212) 777-4900

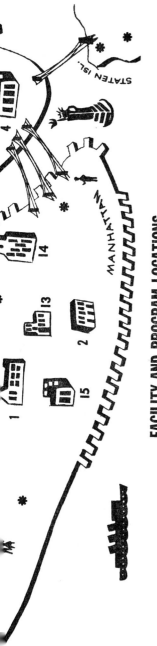

FACILITY AND PROGRAM LOCATIONS

Employment and Guidance Services

1. 215 Park Avenue South
   New York, N.Y. 10003 • 777-4900

Vocational Rehabilitation Facilities

2. 62 West 14 Street
   New York, N.Y. 10011 • 255-4402
3. 2432 Grand Concourse
   Bronx, N.Y. 10458 • 298-4500
4. 1622 Mermaid Avenue
   Brooklyn, N.Y. 11224 • 449-7900

Institutional Workshop Facilities

5. Beth Abraham Hospital
   612 Allerton Avenue
   Bronx, N.Y. 10467
6. Daughters of Jacob Geriatric Center
   167 Street and Findlay Avenue
   Bronx, N.Y. 10456
7. Jewish Institute of Geriatric Care
   271-11 76th Avenue
   New Hyde Park, N.Y. 11040

Neighborhood Manpower Centers

8. 2432 Grand Concourse
   Bronx, N.Y. 10458 • 733-3400
9. 5024 Ft. Hamilton Parkway
   Brooklyn, N.Y. 11219 • 633-3000
10. 222 Division Avenue
    Brooklyn, N.Y. 11211 • 387-3400
11. 97-29 64th Road
    Rego Park, N.Y. 11374 • 275-6700

Skills Training Centers

12. 5013 10th Avenue
    Brooklyn, N.Y. 11219 • 633-3000
13. 510 Sixth Avenue
    New York, N.Y. 10011 • 255-4402
14. 305 Broadway
    New York, N.Y. 10013 • 349-2260
15. 28 East 21st Street
    New York, N.Y. 10010 • 255-4402
16. 555 Remsen Avenue
    Brooklyn, N.Y. 11236 • 342-1300

Special Projects

17. FEGS—Hillside Hospital Drug Project
    Hillside Medical Center
    270-05 76th Avenue
    New Hyde Park, N.Y. 11043 • 343-6700

✱ Other Facilities

The Agency also operates programs out of 26 other locations throughout the New York metropolitan area including family and children agencies, hospitals, community centers, schools, and universities.

individual after he is placed on a job in order to continue the vocational rehabilitation process which never ends since an individual's ability to learn and to improve himself as well as to be able to take on more responsibility is a continuous process, even if that individual is continuing to age chronologically. Yesterday's clerk can become, with the proper supportive services, tomorrow's bookkeeper. The feeling held by many that the elderly and aged have only ten to twelve years to work and therefore can fill a low level job and have no need for advancement is taking from these individuals their God-given right to dignity, to hope and to strive to improve one's lot in life. We are sure that practitioners and administrators, looking at the field of vocational rehabilitation of the disabled elderly and aged population, would agree that no one has the right or the desire to take these basic rights away from the handicapped elderly and aged.

Since there is such a large number of handicapped elderly and aged individuals, this probably would be vastly increased if and when we were to accept the premise that all elderly and aged should be entitled to vocational rehabilitation services since age in itself could be considered a disabling condition.

When we consider the enormity of the problem, the numbers of individuals involved requiring services, the lack of vocational rehabilitation services available for this population, we realize an obligation on the part of the vocational rehabilitation field and of those practitioners and administrators who work in that field to become involved in finding out what services, if any, are available in their communities for serving the elderly handicapped and aged. If these services are not available or are severely limited, they should take on an advocacy role with the public agencies, with the voluntary agencies, and with the community at large to attempt to establish such services for this group.

REFERENCES*

Ayers, G. E., and Mahan, S. P.: A sheltered workshop meets authentic needs of the chronically disabled. *Hospitals, 41:*103-108, 1967.

Background and Issues: Income. Washington, D. C., White House Conference on Aging, 1971.

---

* This reference section was developed for the FEGS Rehabilitation Section of the White House Conference on Aging by Dr. Herbert Rusalem.

Barkin, S.: Concluding address. In *The Employment of Older Workers— Final Report.* Paris, Organization for Economic Cooperation and Development, 1966.

Barshop, I.: Special considerations in providing long-term sheltered workshop experiences for older disabled persons. *Journal of Jewish Communal Service, 41-4:*378-383, 1965.

Baxt, R.: Vocational rehabilitation for the older disabled worker. *Journal of Jewish Communal Service, 37:*309-314, 1961.

Baxt, R.: Vocational rehabilitation of the older disabled worker—A successful program. *Report: Conference on the Rehabilitation of the Older Disabled Worker—The Academician's Responsibility.* Washington, D. C., U. S. Department of Health, Education, and Welfare, 1963.

Belbin, R. M.: Implications for retirement of recent studies on age and working capacity. In Carp, F. M. (Ed.): *The Retirement Process: Report of a Conference,* Gaithersburg, Md. Washington, D. C., U. S. Government Printing Office, 1966, pp. 43-51.

Brant, B.: Employment problems of older disabled workers. In Muthard, J. E. and Morris, W. M. (Eds.): *Counseling the Older Disabled Worker.* Iowa City, Iowa University, 1961, pp. 99-107.

Brotman, H. B.: Counting the aged poor. *Aging,* 3:10-12, April, 1967.

Carp, F. M. (Ed.): Summary and prospect. In *The Retirement Process: Report of a Conference,* Gaithersburg, Md. Bethesda, National Institute of Child Health and Human Development, 1966, pp. 151-160.

Carroll, B.: *Job Satisfaction.* Ithaca, New York State School of Industries and Labor Relations, Cornell University, 1969

Cole, W. E.: Implications for Action in Tennessee. In Holbert, W. M. (Ed.): *Proceedings: Institute on Rehabilitation of the Aging.* Knoxville, University of Tennessee. Washington, D. C., Social and Rehabilitation Service, p. 131-133.

Council Workshop for Senior Citizens Report. New York, National Council of Jewish Women, 1968.

Cumming, E., and Henry, W. E.: *Growing Old.* New York, Basic Books, 1961.

Davis, G. E.: Getting the university and community to work together on problems of the older disabled worker. *Report: Conference on the Rehabilitation of the Older Disabled Worker—The Academician's Responsibility.* Washington, D. C., U. S. Department of Health, Education, and Welfare, 1963.

Draper, J. E. et al.: *Work Attitudes and Retirement Adjustment.* Madison, University of Wisconsin Graduate School of Business, Bureau of Business Research and Service, 1967.

Donahue, W.: Research in the university on the older disabled worker. *Report: Conference on the Rehabilitation of the Older Disabled Worker— The Academician's Responsibility.* Washington, D. C., U. S. Department of Health, Education, and Welfare, 1963.

Elmore, J. L.: Health and rehabilitation of the older person. In Holbert, W. M. (Ed.): *Proceedings: Institute on Rehabilitation of the Aging.* Knoxville, University of Tennessee. Washington, D. C., Social and Rehabilitation Service, pp. 32-42.

Feintuch, A.: Case studies from a generic workshop. *J Rehabil*, 25:15-17, 1959.

Friedrichs, H.: The problem of the older worker in industry. In *The Employment of Older Workers—Final Report*. Paris, Organization for Economic Cooperation and Development, 1966.

Gentry, D. E.: The employer assesses the older worker. In Holbert, W. M. (Ed.): *Proceedings: Institute on Rehabilitation of the Aging.* Knoxville, University of Tennessee. Washington, D. C., Social and Rehabilitation Service, pp. 81-88.

The golden years . . . A tarnished myth. *The Project FIND Report*, Washington, D. C., National Council on the Aging, 1970.

Goldsamt, M. R.: Life satisfaction and the older disabled worker. *J Am Geriatr Soc*, 15:394-399, 1967.

Goodstein, L. D.: Counseling the older worker. In Muthard, J. E. and Morris, W. M. (Eds.): *Counseling the Older Disabled Worker*. Iowa City, University of Iowa, 1961, pp. 78-84.

Gordon, M. S.: Work patterns and retirement. In Kleemeier, R. W. (Ed.): *Aging and Leisure*. New York, Oxford University Press, 1961.

Griew, S.: *Redesigning Jobs for Older Workers*. Paris, Organization for Economic Cooperation and Development, 1964.

Governor's Commission on the Employment and Retirement Problems of Older Workers. Berkeley, The Commission, 1960.

Hanford, J. M. and Evangelos, P.: Rehabilitation of the aged in a mental hospital. *Geriatrics*, 17:809-814, 1962.

Hunter, W. W.: *Preparation for Retirement*. Ann Arbor, Institute of Gerontology, University of Michigan, 1969.

Industrial Gerontology: An Annotated Bibliography on Industrial Change and Aging in the Work Force. Washington, D. C., National Council on the Aging, 1968.

Kaufer, H.: *The Older Handicapped Worker: A Project Report*. St. Louis, Jewish Employment and Vocational Service, 1970.

Kelman, H. R.: An experiment in the rehabilitation of nursing home patients. *Public Health Reports*, 77:356-366, 1962.

Kreps, J. M.: *Lifetime Allocation of Work and Leisure*. Research Report No. 22, Washington, D. C., U. S. Social Security Administration, Office of Research and Statistics, 1968.

Larson, D. C.: Full circle—and more; working with the older age group. *J Rehabil*, 26:15-19, 34-35, 1960.

Leshner, S. S.: Teaching oldsters to develop good work personalities. *Rehabil Rec*, 4:6-8, 1963.

Logan, B. C.: A department store assesses the older worker. In Holbert, W. M. (Ed.): *Proceedings: Institute on Rehabilitation of the Aging,* Knoxville, University of Tennessee. Washington, D. C., Social and Rehabilitation Service, 1967, pp. 73-80.

Mainstream Transforms Aging Colorado Miners Into Skilled Workers. Washington, D. C., U. S. Department of Labor, 1967.

Malikin, D.: *The Satisfaction of Client Needs in a Vocational Rehabilitation Program for Older, Handicapped Workers.* Paper presented at Annual Convention of the American Personnel and Guidance Association, Washington, D. C., 1966.

Mangum, R. J.: *The Human Rights Law and the Older Worker.* Albany, New York State Division of Human Rights, 1969.

Margolin, R., and Goldin, G. (Eds.): *Curriculum Materials Developed from a Conference on Dynamic Programming in the Rehabilitation of the Aging.* Boston, Northeastern University, 1967.

Merriman, I. C.: *Employment After Retirement.* Washington, D. C., U. S. Department of Health, Education, and Welfare, 1967.

Meyers, I.: Seniors find jobs for other seniors. *Harvest Years,* 7:14-18, 1967.

Miller, A. P.: *Programming for the Older Disabled Worker.* Presented at 15th Institute for Rehabilitation Personnel. Carbondale, Southern Illinois University, 1968.

Morris, W. W.: The meaning of work to the older person. In Muthard, J. E. (Ed.): *Counseling the Older Disabled Worker.* Iowa City, University of Iowa, 1961, pp. 69-77.

Moses, D. V., and Lake, C. S.: Geriatrics in the baccalaureate nursing curriculum. *Nursing Outlook,* 16:41-43, 1968.

Odell, C. E.: A comprehensive human resources development program for middle aged and older Americans. In Holbert, W. M. (Ed.): *Proceedings: Institute on Rehabilitation of the Aging,* Knoxville, University of Tennessee. Washington, D. C., Social and Rehabilitation Service, pp. 61-72.

Ondrey, T. R.: Experience diversified. *Employment Service Review, 1:*13-15, 1964.

Orbach, H. L. *et al.: Trends in Early Retirement.* Ann Arbor, Institute of Gerontology, University of Michigan, 1969.

Ortale, L.: Effective placement procedures with older clients. In Muthard, J. E. (Ed.): *Counseling the Older Disabled Worker.* Iowa City, University of Iowa, 1961, pp. 107-119.

Ostfeld, A. M.: Frequency and nature of health problems of retired persons. In Carp, F. M. (Ed.): *The Retirement Process: Report of a conference.* Gaithersburg, Md. Washington, D. C., U. S. Government Printing Office, 1966, p. 83-96.

Page, W. J., Jr.: Resources, problems and potentials of older Americans. In

Holbert, W. M. (Ed.): *Proceedings: Institute on Rehabilitation of the Aging*, Knoxville, University of Tennessee. Washington, D. C., Social and Rehabilitation Service, pp. 8-21.

Pastalan, L. A.: Environmental elements and the physically disabled elderly: Some preliminary findings. In Holbert, W. M. (Ed.): *Proceedings: Institute on Rehabilitation of the Aging*. Knoxville, University of Tennessee. Washington, D. C., Social and Rehabilitation Service, pp. 124-130.

Pastalan, L. A., Perceived needs and differential functions of retirement housing. In Holbert, W. M. (Ed.): *Proceedings: Institute on Rehabilitation of the Aging*. Knoxville, University of Tennessee. Washington, D. C., Social and Rehabilitation Service, pp. 43-60.

Pearlman, E.: A cooperative sheltered workshop program with old age homes. *Journal of Jewish Communal Service*, 37:315-318, 1961.

President's Council on Aging. Employment. In *A Time of Progress for Older Americans*—1965-1966-1967 Report. Washington, D. C., The Council, 1967.

Project for 50's. Cleveland, National Council on the Aging, Welfare Federation of Cleveland, 1966.

Rehabilitation for the Aging, A Growing Responsibility. Washington, D. C., National Rehabilitation Association Committee on Aging, 1960.

The Rehabilitation of the Older Disabled Worker: Proceedings of a Conference. Gainesville, University of Florida, 1964.

Rehabilitation of the Older Disabled Worker: Proceedings of a Conference. West Virginia Vocational Rehabilitation Division, West Virginia Rehabilitation Center Institute. In conjunction with Washington, D. C., U. S. Department of Health, Education, and Welfare, 1964.

Reingold, J.: Octogenarians work for a living in three-year health-morale study. *Hospitals*, 38:59-65, 1964.

Research and Demonstrations Brief. U. S. Social and Rehabilitation Service. *Rehabilitating the Older Disabled Worker: Summary of Final Report.* Washington, D. C., The Service, 1969.

Roberts, S. H.: Tennessee and its aging population: Challenge and opportunity. In Holbert, W. M. (Ed.): *Proceedings: Institute on Rehabilitation of the Aging*. Knoxville, University of Tennessee. Washington, D. C., Social and Rehabilitation Service, pp. 22-31.

Rose, G., Kiwanis senior opportunity program. *Rehabil Rec, 4*:9-11, 1963.

Rudd, J. L., and Feingold, S. N.: Medical and vocational operation in a geriatric workshop. *J Am Geriatr Soc, 7*:349-359, 1959.

Rusalem, H.: Deterrents to vocational disengagement among older workers. *Gerontologist, 3*:64-68, 1963.

Rusalem, H.: Disability, old age and employment. *Journal of Occupational Medicine, 3*:575-578, 1963.

Rusalem, H.: The floundering period in the late careers of older disabled workers. *Rehabil Lit, 24*:34-40, 1963.

Rusalem, H.: Placeability of older disabled clients. *Vocational Guidance Quarterly, 10*:38-41, 1961.

Rusalem, H.: Program for the older disabled worker. *J Rehabil, 25*:24-25, 38-40, 1959.

Rusalem, H.: The prototype: Success story for the aging. *Rehabil Rec,* 1963.

Rusalem, H.: *The Vocational Adjustment of the Older Disabled Worker: A Selective Review of the Recent Literature.* New York, Federation Employment and Guidance Service, 1967.

Rusalem, H.: The Vocational Potentialities of Older Disabled Persons Who Resist Retirement. Paper presented at the VI World Congress of Gerontology, Copenhagen, Denmark, 1963.

Rusalem, H. *et al.*: Neighborhood rehabilitation for the aged. *Rehabil Rec,* 7:28-31, 1966.

Rusalem, H., Baxt, R., and Barshop, I.: *The Vocational Rehabilitation of Older Handicapped Workers.* Final Report. New York, Federation Employment and Guidance Service, 1963.

Rusalem, H., Baxt, R., and Barshop, I.: *Rehabilitating the Older Disabled Worker.* Final Report. New York, Federation Employment and Guidance Service, 1967.

Rusalem, H., Baxt, R., and Barshop, I.: *The Vocational Rehabilitation of Neighborhood-Bound Older Disabled Persons: A Program Guide.* New York, Federation Employment and Guidance Service, 1967.

Rusalem, H., and Dill, S.: Vocational rehabilitation of the older, disabled person. *J Rehabil, 27*:19-20, 1961.

Schupack, M. B.: Research on employment problems of older workers. *Gerontologist, 2*:157-163, 1962.

Schweisheimer, W.: Older workers in industry. *Supervision,* January, 1967, pp. 24-25.

A Sheltered Workshop at the Home for Jewish Aged. Report of the Committee on Services to the Aged. Kansas City, Jewish Vocational Services, 1953.

Slavick, F.: *Compulsory and Flexible Retirement in the American Economy.* Ithaca, New York, Cornell University, School of Industrial and Labor Relations, 1966.

Sobel, I., and Wilcock, R. C.: *Placement Techniques for Older Workers.* Organization for Economic Cooperation and Development, Paris, 1966.

Stahler, A.: Significance of manpower retraining for rehabilitation of the older disabled worker. *Report: Conference on the Rehabilitation of the Older Disabled Worker—The Academician's Responsibility.* Washington, D. C., U. S. Department of Health, Education, and Welfare, 1963.

Strum, H. M.: Job redesign for older workers. *Bulletin No. 1523.* Washington, D. C., U. S. Department of Labor, 1967.

The Therapeutic Workshop for Older Persons: Final Report. Chicago, Jewish Vocational Service, 1967.

Training and Employment of the Older Worker. Recent Findings and Recommendations on Older Worker Experimental and Demonstration Projects. Washington, D. C., U. S. Department of Labor, U. S. Manpower Administration, 1968.

Vocational Rehabilitation of Handicapped Persons Over 60 Years of Age. Unpublished, Milwaukee, Jewish Vocational Service, 1964.

Walker, R. A.: The use of rehabilitation centers for the older worker. In Muthard, J. E. (Ed.): *Counseling the Older Disabled Worker.* Iowa City, University of Iowa, 1961, pp. 61-68.

Woll, W.: Functional capacities of the older disabled worker. *Report: Conference on the Rehabilitation of the Older Disabled Worker—The Academician's Responsibility.* Washington, D. C., U. S. Department of Health, Education, and Welfare, 1963.

Work Evaluation, Training and Placement Project for Older Disabled Workers. Kansas City, Jewish Vocational Service, 1964.

Zamir, L. J.: *Expanding Dimensions in Rehabilitation.* Springfield, Thomas, 1969.

PART III

Working With the Physically Disabled

CHAPTER 8

SERVING THE BLIND AND THE VISUALLY IMPAIRED IN A REHABILITATION FACILITY

HERBERT RUSALEM and HAROLD RICHTERMAN

REHABILITATION HAD ITS BEGINNINGS in the United States in 1840 with the establishment of the first sheltered workshop for the blind by Dr. Samuel Gridley Howe at the Perkins School for the Blind in Boston, Massachusetts. Throughout the nineteenth century, rehabilitation programs for this client group were established in many communities to provide blind* people with opportunities for work, self-development, and strategies and devices for overcoming the barriers imposed upon them by visual loss. Early in the twentieth century, commissions and other types of state agencies for the blind began to appear, offering more comprehensive, multiple function programs that contained preventive, educational, and rehabilitative service components. By the time that the Federal-State Vocational Rehabilitation Program was launched in 1920, a functional network of agencies for the blind was already engaged in the difficult process of assisting blind persons to make a place for themselves in the sighted world (Farrell, 1956). Indeed, as the years went by and general rehabilitation programs proliferated, attempts were made to achieve fiscal and social advantages by combining parallel general and blind rehabilitation programs into single service entities. Although the matter received wide discussion and although a number of attempts were made to merge the two approaches, the rehabilitation picture of the 1970's still finds a large majority of blind persons being rehabilitated through special agencies, divisions, and programs developed exclusively for this client group.

---

* Blind is defined as 20/200 or less in the better eye with optimum correction or a limitation in the visual field that subtends an angle of 20 degrees or less,

The current rehabilitation status of special rehabilitation programs for the blind can be described in these terms (Rusalem, 1973):

a. A majority of the fifty states maintain separate state rehabilitation agencies for the blind. The others operate a single state rehabilitation agency for both groups in which separate divisions or programs for blind clients exist within the orbit of their general programs.

b. With few exceptions blind persons receiving sheltered workshop rehabilitation service do so through facilities affiliated with National Industries for the Blind.

c. Most of the major rehabilitation advances for blind persons had their origins in special programs for the blind. Among these are the Talking Book, low vision aids, mobility training, instruction in personal management, training in computer and other new occupations for the blind, and intensive selective placement in community employment.

d. In the absence of firm data bearing on the matter, most administrators of programs for the blind express the conviction that blind persons are not served as effectively by general as by specialized rehabilitation agencies. Their belief is that blind persons tend to get "lost in the cracks" of general agencies and do not receive the intensive and specialized assistance that they need. They hold that this is so because blind clients tend to have a low priority in such agencies, specially trained personnel are not available to help them, special training equipment is lacking, and the special rehabilitation approaches they need are not available.

The philosophical question about whether blind persons should be served by agencies dealing exclusively with the problems of blindness has been argued back and forth for generations. Those who favor a specialized approach feel that there are identifiable attributes of blindness that require specialized methods and facilities and that general rehabilitation workers are not equipped with the interest, training or disposition to provide blind persons with the specialized forms of assistance they need. On the other hand, those who favor incorporation of blind clients into general rehabilitation agency caseloads find it paradoxical that while the integration of blind persons into sighted society is accepted in principle, extreme service segregation is actually being practiced. Furthermore, they believe that those who specialized in segregated service to blind persons are prisoners of an obsolete tradition which reflects medieval notions about blindness. Although this controversy is an interesting and significant one, the fact remains that most blind persons currently receive rehabilitation service from specialized agencies and that, unless a dramatic change occurs in our rehabilitation service delivery system, this will continue to be the case. Advocates of specialization of service argue that segregation is necessary to prepare blind persons for subsequent integration.

In this respect, it is important to note that service rehabilitation also is supported by existing legislation (Hardy and Cull, 1972). For example:

a. The federal vocational rehabilitation acts grant each state the option of maintaining two separate rehabilitation programs —one for the blind and another for other disability groups. In response to this provision, a majority of the states have opted for specialized rehabilitation agencies for the blind.

b. The Javits-Wagner-O'Day Act, insuring special treatment workshops for the disabled in government purchases of selected products, mandates (after federal prisons) priorities for workshops for the blind as compared to workshops for other disability groups. Indeed, the original Wagner-O'Day Act was restricted in its benefits exclusively to workshops serving blind persons.

c. Blind persons receive special economic benefits under federal legislation, including income tax exemptions, free mailing privileges, special rates on common carriers, and a special status under welfare and social security programs.

d. A well-established network of specialized agencies for the blind continues to take leadership in legislative matters relating to blind persons under the leadership of such strong groups as National Industries for the Blind, the American Foundation for the Blind, and the American Association of Workers for the Blind.

In brief, specialized agencies for the blind now dominate the field and there are no current indications that they soon will be

displaced (Rusalem, 1968). In practice, when a sound specialized agency exists in a community, the probability is that almost
all of the blind persons in that community will be served in that
program rather than in a general one. The other side of the coin
is that blind persons in a community tend to receive services
from general agencies only when strong specialized programs are
not available. Historically, rehabilitation agencies for the blind
have shown remarkable durability despite efforts to replace them
with general programs. The stability of these agencies over the
decades suggests that factors in addition to their history, tradition, and status in the rehabilitation establishment are at work.
Specialized agencies form a powerful advocacy system for their
own preservation as well as for the interests of blind persons;
American legislators see a logic in specialized services; the agencies for the blind are achieving many of their objectives, and
the system is too valuable to be dismantled. Therefore, it may
be concluded that specialized agencies for the blind continue to
fill a vital function in American society and that their replace-
ment by general programs is not imminent in most communities.

The role of the specialized rehabilitation agency seems to
spring from the unique quality of blindness as a disability. Although each disability differs from the others in important respects, the differences that inhere in blindness appear to be of
such a magnitude that they require highly specialized interventions, personnel, equipment, and the facilities that cannot ordinarily be contained within the framework of most general
agencies for the handicapped. In exceptional cases, these differences are being managed in general rehabilitation programs. For
example, blind persons are receiving certain services from general agency programs in cities such as Syracuse, New York, and in
states like Wisconsin. But whether the delivery of comprehensive
rehabilitation services to the blind is possible even in these agencies is still a moot point.

Special Characteristics of the Blindness Experience

Crucial to the argument that special rehabilitation facilities
are required for blind persons is the contention that the blind
experience differs from other disability experiences. The litera-

ture abounds in evidence that it is so. One of the most definitive statements on this point was made by Father Thomas J. Carroll (1961) who identified twenty specific disabling losses that are imposed upon one by the onset of blindness. These losses are so pervasive and all encompassing that they penetrate almost every area of living and, indeed, represent in their totality a massive reduction in one's capacity to cope with the social and physical environment. In earlier statements Lowenfeld (1950) stressed the significant losses in mobility, control of oneself in the world, and environmental control that accompany blindness. As in Carroll's case, the losses described by Lowenfeld are so massive in character that they divest the affected individual of vital attributes and functions. Essentially, the wide-ranging deficits suffered by blind persons would appear to be the following:

1. Limitations in mobility.
2. Limitations in awareness and control of the environment.
3. Limitations on communication capabilities.
4. Limitations in appreciation of the world about one in all its beauty and diversity.
5. Limitations in cognitive abilities and learning.
6. Limitations in achieving acceptance of one's self as a relatively normal person in our society.
7. Limitation in educational, recreational, and vocational activities.
8. Limitations imposed upon one by labeling.

When blind persons appear on the threshold of a rehabilitation agency, it will be noted that they probably possess one or more of the following specific problems (Chevigny and Braverman, 1950):

a. Their mobility is so restricted that they depend heavily upon others for travel assistance.

b. Relatively few stimulus signals reach them, especially in the visual area. Since visual stimuli are by far the most informative of all communicators of environmental conditions, dangers, and opportunities, they lack reliable current information about essential features of the world around them. This inadequate data base reduces their capacity to cope with, and control, the environment. Since they are likely to make decisions on the basis of erroneous or incomplete inputs, their responses are less positive and parsimonious.

c. Whole areas of communication are partitioned off from them, including most daily newspapers, magazines, books, the visual parts of television programs, observations, films, and demonstrations. In some cases, the blockage is partial so that they can attend to the audio of television or read recorded magazines, but vision is such a dominant sense that what is left after it is excluded can be very incomplete and unsatisfying. Communication problems also exist in face to face communications, attendance at lectures, group experiences, and casual conversations especially when facial expressions and gestures are used to convey subtlety, meaning, and direction.

d. Aesthetic experiences are restricted. Much that is enjoyable in this world is visual—two dimensional art, photographs, drawings, scenic views, motion pictures, the visual impact of a stage presentation or a musical performance, and the faces of one's loved ones. Deprived of these experiences, blind persons lose vast areas of aesthetic pleasure and appreciation.

e. Knowledge may be outdated in a fast-moving technological society; survival and advancement often hinge upon uninterrupted learning. Although it need not be so, the reality is that most learning stimuli require an unimpaired visual channel. For example, most updating information is transmitted through books, journals, newspapers, magazines, bulletins, drawings, charts, maps, manuals, films, billboards, posters, television, and observations. To the extent that auditory and tactile media cannot replace graphics, sightless individuals are isolated from vital sources of learning and, in the process, fall hopelessly behind other people in keeping pace with new development and essential changes that are constantly occurring in the community.

f. Their capacities are held in low regard. Physical difference in our society still is only partially accepted. Even at this late date in our history, blindness often is perceived by many sighted persons as such a catastrophic condition that even the smallest degree of independence is considered inconceivable within the boundaries of the disability. Large segments of the public still consider all blind people to be helpless and to have generalized unrelated disorders that extend far beyond the inability to see. For example, many blind persons continue to be viewed as objects of commiseration, pity, overwhelming protectiveness, and shelter. In daily experience, the essential humanity of most blind persons is overshadowed by a distorted sense of difference and incapacity that prevails at every social, economic, and cultural level.

g. Blind persons are victims of social prejudice. Although a visual limitation in and of itself, if blind persons are deprived of numerous opportunities because of the inability to respond to visual stimuli, the dimensions of disadvantage are extended unreasonably by the erroneous perceptions and biases of the gatekeepers of this country. Thus, although blind people can function well in many activities, they are denied opportunities to do so because unenlightened non-disabled people bar the threshold and arbitrarily exclude them from entry into self-fulfilling situations. Paradoxically, those among the non-disabled who mourn most piously for the losses suffered by blind persons sometimes are among the quickest to exaggerate these losses by denying blind persons reasonable social and vocational opportunities. For example, for many years blind persons were denied employment in general state rehabilitation agencies, presumably because of their inability to drive an automobile in their field work.

h. Like other minority groups, blind individuals are often viewed in class terms. That is, they are mistakenly considered to have certain characteristics in common, yet, all but one of these perceived commonalities have no basis in fact. The one exception is that all blind persons have seriously impaired vision or no vision at all. All other perceived group similarities in personality, intellectual ability, response systems, understanding, independence, and motivation are nonexistent products of misinformation and unsupported bias. Yet, as a consequence of this bias, blind persons are routinely deprived of their individuality and thoughtlessly classified under a label that connotes helplessness to key decision makers.

In summary, the blindness experience for most people adds up to a massive psychological, physical, social, educational, and vocational deprivation. In actuality, there are few, if any, compensations to being blind. On the contrary, blindness affects a person's fundamental skills, inputs, understandings, controls, and comprehensions, reducing in almost all cases the capacity to do things as sighted people do them. Although blindness is not nearly as handicapping as most non-disabled people believe, it is still one of the most limitating of all disabilities.

The vast network of specialized facilities that society has established for the rehabilitation and nurturance of blind persons gives testimony to the perceived number and severity of deficits that customarily result from blindness (Lukoff and Whiteman, undated). The continued existence and continued expansion of such programs reflects the hopeful belief that these deficits are not necessarily immutable, hopeless, or so overreaching that rehabilitation is impossible. Indeed, the reverse is true. Hundreds of thousands of blind persons have been helped by increasingly sophisticated techniques to achieve higher levels of community functioning, despite multiple problems. In fact, successful rehabilitation is occurring to thousands of multi-handicapped blind persons whose blindness is accompanied by hearing loss, mental retardation, advancing age, emotional disturbance, physical health problems, social and cultural disadvantage, cognitive and learning difficulties aggravated by sustained isolation, and neurological conditions that manifest themselves in vast areas of impaired human response.

Although the controversy concerning the suitability of blind persons for rehabilitation service at general agencies will continue for many years to come, some aspects of the problem are already settled. That is, it is thought that blind persons who are relatively intact in every way other than their blindness may be able, under certain conditions, to function successfully in a rehabilitation environment engineered primarily for sighted persons. Although the precise size of this more competent blind subgroup is not known, the maximum could conservatively be put at some 5 percent or fewer of the adult blind population. On the other hand, it is now pretty well accepted that blind persons at the other extreme—the aged, the multi-disabled, and poorly-equipped—require specialized programming at least initially in their rehabilitation experience. The number of individuals in this less capable blind group is very large, since more than half of all blind persons are sixty-five years of age and over and, perhaps, an additional 25 to 40 percent of the remainder has complicating problems other than in vision that, in and of themselves, would render them eligible for state rehabilitation service. The middle group, some 5 to 20 percent really are the targets of the facilities controversy since both the general and the specialized agencies perceive them as potential clients.

Essential Requirements of a Rehabilitation Program for Blind Persons

Viewed in the context of the nature of the blindness experience and the special rehabilitation problems that blind persons present, it is evident that members of this group need the range of services usually offered to clients with other disabilities, including medical, social, psychological, educational and vocational evaluations, individual and group counseling, personal adjustment and skills training, educational and vocational placement, recreation and group work, community organization and advocacy, vocational follow through, and long-range career guidance (Malikin and Rusalem, 1969). The difference is that they need to receive these general services with special reference to the impact of visual loss upon rehabilitation programming, a variable that necessitates certain service modifications and the addition of selected specialized intervention into the rehabilitation service.

Adapting customary services, such as counseling and training, in order to make them more suitable for blind persons, can be a challenge to general and special rehabilitation workers. In counseling, for example, it is necessary for the counselor to be conscious of the meaning of blindness to the individual, the techniques of communicating with people who cannot see, the influence of experience deprivation on the person's relatedness and sense of reality, and the pervasive, deleterious effects of negative public attitudes toward blindness. Similarly, in the evaluation process, assessment tasks should be selected for their relevance to those who cannot see and administered under performance standards that are meaningful for blind individuals. Furthermore, in providing rehabilitation training to the visually impaired person, agency personnel should be aware of the special learning styles of blind individuals and should modify instructional procedures accordingly.

In effect, customary rehabilitation procedures, while generally applicable to blind clients, need to be adapted, sometimes radically, to make them applicable to individuals with seriously defective vision (Hardy and Cull, 1972). Thus, any agency, general or specialized, that plans to serve members of this group must examine all customary agency procedures, assess their compatibility with the blindness experience, and systematically modify them to fit the situation. This approach is not unfamiliar to rehabilitation agencies since modifications customarily are made in meeting the special needs of the mentally retarded, the physically limited or the emotionally disabled. In fact, many rehabilitation agencies, both general and specialized, have had considerable experience in making such alterations. However, it should be kept in mind that modifications made for blind clients tend to be relatively extensive and to lie outside the customary service of general agency personnel. Beyond these program modifications, agencies serving blind clients will have to initiate a group of services that have no close counterpart in general rehabilitation programming since they relate specifically to the blindness experience and, generally, do not apply to clients with normal levels of visual functioning. Some of the special programming provisions are listed below (Rusalem, 1973).

Vision Rehabilitation

It is obvious that a rehabilitation agency serving blind persons should have access to ophthalmological resources, to other medical specialities, and that comprehensive functionally oriented eye examinations should be routinely conducted for all blind clients. In addition, it should be noted that many blind clients require the special services of a vision rehabilitation facility. At such a center, the characteristics of residual vision are studied intensively, remedial procedures are prescribed and administered, and suitable aids are fitted and adapted to individual need. Omission of this step in the rehabilitation process for blind persons violates the principle of eliminating or alleviating correctable impairments prior to long-range rehabilitation planning and programming. The fact is that 10 to 20 percent or more of the blind persons who enter rehabilitation programs of any kind can benefit from special low-vision services. Such services are delivered in some cases by medical facilities which have the advantage of access to all corollary needed medical resources that may be needed conjunctively by a blind individual. In other cases, low-vision rehabilitation is conducted through programs sponsored by agencies for the blind that have the advantage of close coordination with other rehabilitation services and a broader use of skilled specialized optometrists who, unfortunately, may be accorded only a subsidiary role, if any, in hospital-based programs. Essential in such a program is an appropriate training service that instructs the blind person in the most efficacious means of adapting to, and using, the aids that are prescribed for him. This is an indispensable, highly technical specialization to which even well-established agencies for the blind ordinarily lack access.

Health Evaluation and Health Care.

Most rehabilitation agencies use their own or nearby health resources to assess the current state of the blind client's general health and suggest procedures that will maintain or restore satisfactory health levels. The special need in this area in relation to blindness is for a medical staff that recognizes the interplay between certain physical conditions such as diabetes, the aging process, malnutrition, and circulatory problems and visual performance and the preventive and therapeutic interventions that are necessary to maximize and preserve a blind person's residual visual efficiency. Contrary to expectations, many physicians, including ophthalmologists, are not as well informed as they should be about the relationship between general health and eye health and the steps that should be taken to insure the most favorable visual response of every blind individual who has residual sight.

Restoration in Other Sensory and Health Areas

Some rehabilitation programs for blind individuals become preoccupied with the blindness component in the client's life. Although the loss of vision does result in challenging problems for the affected individual and those who serve him, the blind are subject to all the other health limitations that occur to people in general. Thus, blindness does not exempt a person from deficits in physical health, hearing, speech, intellectual ability, mental health, or neurological problems. When combined disabilities do appear, they can be more overwhelming and far more serious than the sum of the two or more conditions concerned. For example, many of the strategies developed by blind persons to cope with their problems depend upon the use of their hearing, intelligence, alertness, eye-body coordination, and physical vigor. Reductions in any or all of these areas are extremely serious. Thus, all aspects of blind person's health and, if possible, restoration should be provided whenever a health condition imposes additional losses on the individual.

Psychological Testing

Most psychological testing instruments present visual stimuli to the subject and compare his performance on them with norms developed from a sample of sighted persons. In view of the visual demand and comparisons found in such instruments, they should be used with great caution and skill with blind persons and, unless suitable adaptations are made in their administration, scoring, and interpretation, the results of testing will have limited meaning for the rehabilitation team and the blind client. It is apparent that psychologists who examine blind clients should have had special training and ample experience in working with this group so that they are equipped to adjust standard procedures and arrive at reasonably accurate assessments of the intelligence, personality, aptitudes, and interests of blind rehabilitation clients. Beyond this is the fact that research activities conducted since World War II have produced special testing instruments and approaches that are acceptable substitutes for more familiar standardized instruments. Such substitutions are required because more general tests often are grossly inadequate even in the hands of a skilled examiner for measuring the capacities of blind persons. Needless to say, anyone in rehabilitation who is charged with the evaluation of blind persons should know such specialized instruments thoroughly and should be capable of using them skillfully.

Learning Capacities

The pioneering work of Rusalem and Rusalem (1972) in developing innovative approaches to the measurement of learning capacities and in evolving instructional programs to make the fullest possible use of residual learning resources in both disabled and non-disabled persons has general implications for all of rehabilitation, but especially for the blind. In essence, Rusalem and Rusalem have noted that rehabilitation services are instructional in character; that is, in order to achieve rehabilitation goals, handicapped persons are required to learn many new responses. For example, in mastering cane mobility techniques, the effective use of visual aids, and procedures for attending to and using auditory cues, blind people become involved in complex learning situations. Despite this, instruction in these and other vital rehabilitation areas almost always is offered in an intuitive stereotyped fashion by agency personnel who are partially, if at all, informed about individual learning styles and the learning problems of visually limited people. Thus, regardless of his particular learning needs, the blind person is expected to adapt to customary instructional procedures in a rehabilitation center, resulting in a far greater percentage of failure and partial success in the process than should be the case. Although the learning capacities approach developed by Rusalem and Rusalem should be an integral feature in any rehabilitation program, the learning component in rehabilitation continues to be neglected.

Mental Health Services

Blind persons are as subject to mental health problems as all other people. However, it must be recognized that the blind experience introduces special stresses and mental health hazards in the lives of visually limited persons. These additional stresses relate to the difficulties that one has in accepting himself as a blind person and in coping with the differential attitudes and biases of others toward his blindness. As clearly demonstrated by Cholden (1958), the emotional impact of blindness can be catastrophic and extremely damaging to emotional stability. During the past generation, pioneering work by Blank (1957) and others has confirmed the hypothesis that the blind experience precipitates mental health problems that require adapted mental health interventions. Although mental health specialists may not agree on the respective roles of castration, narcissism, organ inferiority, and other psychosocial variables in generating and sustaining emotional problems in blind persons, there is a general consensus that those who deliver mental health services to blind individuals should be cognizant of the potency of visual loss in the emotional area. Furthermore, they should be skillful in using the psychotherapeutic procedures that are required to help people to cope with the intra- and interpersonal emotional sequelae of blindness.

Mobility Instruction

As indicated earlier in this chapter, the loss of mobility that inevitably accompanies blindness is one of the most significant deprivations suffered by blind persons. Unless the client can be taught to travel independently and safely and unless he can be taught to form mental maps of his routes and destinations, all other aspects of his rehabilitation will be deterred. Indeed, the establishment of some level of independent movement often constitutes the key to entry into employment, advancement in educational programs, success in interpersonal relationships, and participation in community affairs. The process of training blind persons in the use of the cane or the guide dog is so technical that special educational programs and facilities have been established just for this purpose. Thus, every blind person who needs this service receives mobility instruction either through qualified personnel employed by a rehabilitation agency for the blind or through a special guide dog training school such as The Seeing Eye.

Self-Care Activities

Serious visual loss usually reduces an individual's capacity to manage commonplace everyday situations such as dressing, care of one's person, personal hygiene, maintenance of clothing, engaging in common activities such as dialing a telephone, eating, making change and the myriad of other daily tasks that others take for granted. Such mundane activities are not mundane at all to the blind person; on the contrary, they require special attention, skills, and strategies which do not develop automatically. Painstaking and professional instruction in this area is required so that the blind person can take the route that is most compatible with his physical capacities and learning style.

Home Responsibilities

Home and family life requires both men and women in American society to assume responsibilities for home-related tasks. Such tasks usually are carried out without fanfare or problems by sighted persons. Yet, lighting a gas stove, preparing a meal, storing foodstuffs for easy retrieval, or keeping the premises clean and in order can be a major challenge when performed without the benefit of full sight. In consideration of the crucial necessity for blind men and women to fill functional roles in the home, rehabilitation programs for this group provide for specialized instruction in homemaking activities. This instruction is built upon special teaching techniques and procedures that are not ordinarily found in general rehabilitation programs, indicating the need for differentiated service in the homemaking area.

Home repairs constitute a closely related program element. Maintaining one's home almost always requires some repair and maintenance work. Do-it-yourself considerations are especially vital when the hiring of others to do the job is costly and when the technical personnel needed in this connection are not readily available. If properly instructed, many blind persons can perform an amazing variety of jobs in the home that contribute to more comfortable family living, including wiring electric appliances, changing faucet washers, hanging shades, curtains, and venetian blinds, installing door locks, making minor repairs, and servicing small appliances. Here again, special instructional procedures are required to help the blind person to learn repair and maintenance techniques despite the effects of blindness and to evolve tactics for coping with tasks that ordinarily are accomplished with the help of sight.

Communication Skills

Many interpersonal and business transactions are conducted through the written word. Since blindness reduces or eliminates inkprint reading and customary handwriting for most blind persons, means should be developed to circumvent this loss. Otherwise, vital connections with the outside world will be severed. This requires selective instruction in Braille, recording techniques, listening skills, writing without vision, typing, and the use of the telephone. Over the years, specialized procedures have been developed for helping blind persons to master these skills. Thus, rehabilitation personnel who serve this group should not only be aware of these procedures, but should be fully qualified to administer them to blind clients.

Vocational Evaluation and Training

Vocational evaluation and skills training in general rehabilitation agencies commonly are conducted via visual demonstrations. That is, the staff member performs the task while the trainee observes him in the process and attempts to duplicate the performance. If instructional aids are used at all, they rely on visual stimuli such as charts, pictures, work sheets, and finished models. Obviously, such techniques have limited value, if any, for blind trainees. The loss of sight requires quite different approaches to be used with this client group. A number of these approaches have been advocated by Richterman (undated) and other specialists in service to the blind, including the "laying of hands" on the blind client, doing a task *with* him through extensive use of tactile and auditory cues. Unless evaluation and training personnel are skilled in the use of these instructional measures and the accompanying training materials that have evolved for those with limited vision, instruction of the client will be difficult, frustrating, and perhaps, counter-productive.

Sheltered Employment Opportunities

Salmon (Zahl, 1950) estimated that fewer than 20 percent of all blind persons qualify for placement in competitive industry because of complicating aging and multi-disability problems. Even within this 20 percent, long-range deprivations, emotional responses to blindness, and public apathy and rejection reduce the probability of placement in industry still further. Therefore, if a majority of blind persons emerging from rehabilitation programs are to enter employment at all, it will have to be under long-term sheltered circumstances. Consequently, rehabilitation programs serving blind persons should have access to a variety of long-term sheltered, as well as competitive, work stations. A broad range of sheltered work situations is especially critical if work-motivated limited blind people are to engage in remunerative employment when opportunities in outside industry are not appropriate or available.

Although the special programming areas noted above do not exhaust the total range of special concerns, they do suggest the gamut of additional provisions that have to be made in delivering rehabilitation service to blind individuals in order to achieve rehabilitation goals. Differentiated offerings will be needed at least in the following: vision rehabilitation, health evaluation and health care, physical restoration, psychological testing, learning capacities, mental health services, mobility instruction, self-care activities, home responsibilities, communication skills, vocational evaluation and training and sheltered employment opportunities. Administratively, arrangements will be required for each of these services:

1. Physical space should be provided to accommodate the pro-

gram. For example, vision rehabilitation requires special clinical areas in which light and other environmental features can be readily altered and controlled.

2. Special equipment devised expressly for, or adapted to, blind persons should be installed. For example, production machines should be properly guarded for those who cannot see and aisles in workshop or training areas should be delineated by proper railings and tactile cues.

3. Social and vocational rehabilitation tasks should be selected and engineered so that they are compatible with, and relevant for, blind persons.

4. Staff members and clients with other disabilities should be helped to accept and work with the visually handicapped.

5. Agency personnel should be trained in the special techniques of serving blind persons.

6. Administrators should be sensitized to the special problems of blind persons. For example, they need to be aware of the fact that the staff-to-client ratio will be smaller than in serving many other disability groups and that the costs of the service probably will be higher. Indeed, in the initial stages of working with the multi-handicapped, such as the deaf-blind, service may need to be delivered on a one-to-one basis.

7. A balance should be achieved between the specialized needs of the blind person to be served in a specialized manner and his concurrent needs to be integrated into a general community environment. Thus, the rehabilitation agency should be able to separate instances in which specialized service is required from those in which integrated activities should be planned so that the blind client's progress toward ultimate absorption into undifferentiated community living will be accelerated.

8. Specially trained personnel should be available in such areas as mobility training, self-care, home responsibilities, communications, vision rehabilitation, and vocational evaluation and training. These personnel should undergo special orientation and training in blindness rehabilitation and

provision should be made for their continuing supervision by specialized personnel who have special skills and experience in serving blind persons.

Agency Setting for Serving Blind Persons

Many general and specialized rehabilitation agencies report that they are successfully serving blind persons. Yet, even a casual review of their programs, personnel, and facilities suggests that they provide only a segment of the requisite services and conditions described in this chapter. Even in their imperfect form, these agencies are making a contribution to the rehabilitation of blind individuals, but this should not be regarded as constituting a comprehensive rehabilitation service for this client group. Agencies that function partialistically with this caseload undoubtedly improve the welfare and status of the blind persons whom they serve, but they also perpetuate areas of serious disability in such clients. For example, a failure to somehow provide routine vision rehabilitation facilities prolongs visual limitations unnecessarily; the inability or unwillingness of an agency to assess, prescribe for, and implement programs that harmonize with a client's learning capacities, subject him to hazard and unwarranted and often disorganizing failure, and agencies that pay little heed to communication skills permit the persistence of weakened links between the client and his human environment. In other words, blindness has to be viewed as a constellation of many different conditions, each of which interacts with the others to form a single handicapping condition. Successful treatment of this disability gestalt demands attention to all of these variables as well as to the condition of blindness, as a whole.

Returning now to the issue of preferred sources of rehabilitation service for blind persons, it becomes evident why many general agencies fail to qualify to serve blind persons in a global sense. In order to satisfy the criteria stipulated in this chapter for rehabilitation programs for blind people, general and specialized agencies are required to make extensive commitments of space, equipment, personnel, administrative resources, and community facilities. Considering the relatively small number of blind persons in any community, the costs of serving them and the unique service components that should be included in comprehensive rehabilitation programs, it is apparent that the required degree of agency commitment is probably beyond the means of most general rehabilitation agencies.

Arrayed against this position are those who believe that segregation by reason of a disability category is generally undesirable. They contend that even if a general agency lacks all the resources needed to fully meet every limitation of blind clients, the deleterious psychosocial effects of any segregation for any purpose, no matter how praiseworthy, are so pernicious that even partially inadequate service resources in general agencies are preferable to segregation. This argument is tenable if, indeed, blind persons do achieve social integration in general programs and if, in fact, the absence of a vital element in the general program is relatively unimportant to ultimate rehabilitation success and if integration, *per se*, is necessarily of greater moment than anything else in the life of a blind person. Some notion of the validity of a rigidly held integration position may be derived from conversations with blind persons, themselves, not all of whom are as enthusiastic about integration as professional workers in general rehabilitation agencies.

Service Delivery Models for Rehabilitating Blind Persons

The following are the major models now being used in American rehabilitation:

The Fully Integrated Model

In this model, blind rehabilitation clients receive all the rehabilitation assistance they need through a facility that serves a variety of disabilities, but which does not maintain a separate department of a differentiated program for blind persons. Generally, this model provides the minimal environmental modifications, special equipment, personnel specialists in service to blind individuals, and specially designed tasks and processes. Although it may be applied to a broad range of blind persons, this model is customarily restricted to blind persons who previously received special services elsewhere or retain considerable residual vision and have relatively few complicating problems.

The Integrated Department Model

In this model, blind persons are served in the framework of a general rehabilitation agency which maintains a special department or differentiated program for the visually handicapped. In some respects, this department is an agency within an agency, with the mini-agency often functioning somewhat autonomously. Under this plan, blind persons may be segregated in the differentiated department or program early in their rehabilitation experience when they need specialized assistance the most. As they make progress, they may be increasingly integrated into other divisions of the general agency service. Commonly, a blind client's program is made up of segregated and some integrated components, both functioning contemporaneously. Advocates of this approach believe that the benefits of both general and specialized services thus accrue to the blind individual.

The Cooperative Agency Model

In this model, general and specialized rehabilitation agencies join forces. At the beginning of the blind client's rehabilitation experience, the specialized agency usually assumes a dominant role, engaging in highly specialized self-care, communications, mobility, and personal adjustment interventions. As time goes by and as client competence and self-acceptance are augmented more, program activities are scheduled at the nearby general agency. Toward the end of his program, the client may be enrolled full time in the general agency. This plan also aims at providing blind persons with the benefits of both the integrated and segregated approaches to rehabilitation service. Sometimes, as in the case of joint programming between the New York State Commission for the Visually Handicapped and the Federation of the Handicapped, the disinclination of the specialized agencies to serve a particular subgroup (in this case, homebound blind persons) necessitates a two-tier approach; the first or the intensive readjustment tier is offered by specialized agency, while subsequent more general service comes through the local integrated agency.

The Community-Based Model

This widely recommended model prepares the blind client for participation in community services for the non-disabled such as family counseling, employment, education, recreation, and socialization. As soon as the client attains a readiness to benefit from such community resources, arrangements are made for him to do so. In time, he may either disengage himself fully from the specialized agency for the blind or reduce the amount of service he receives from it. Since, theoretically, the visually handicapped person is entitled to all the general community services that are available to others who reside in his area, he is not only urged but trained to use them. Although the concept undergirding this model has received considerable acceptance, it has been attained only infrequently in actual practice. At this point, it is difficult to know whether the failures in this regard are due to the weakness of the concept itself, or the inability or unwillingness of general and specialized agencies to implement it properly.

The Temporally Segregated Model

In this model, blind persons receive all or most of their rehabilitation service in a special environment designed expressly for blind persons, with the understanding (as in the case of a state rehabilitation agency for the blind) that the segregated experience has definite time limits. Thus, as soon as the person achieves the rehabilitation goals set with him, his case is closed at the specialized agency and he moves on to other and, hopefully, more integrated community experiences. Presumably, the blind person is prepared during rehabilitation for his subsequent post-rehabilitation integrated experiences. In practice, however, this doesn't always happen. Furthermore, temporally limited programs face the dilemma of what to do with the multi-handicapped and disadvantaged blind person who may need specialized services that extend well beyond case closure, perhaps, indefinitely.

The Long-Term Segregated Model

This model helps the blind client to achieve improved levels of educational, social, vocational, and psychological functioning within a segregated agency setting. After maximum benefit has been derived from the rehabilitation program, the client may be encouraged to establish himself in unsegregated society. In many cases, he will be offered long-term post-rehabilitation opportunities for employment, adult education, recreation, and/or socialization in the segregated agency environment. This service may be offered for a period of years, perhaps, for as long as the client chooses to stay with it. At the turn of the twentieth century, this model was common, and even though it is less in evidence today, it continues with remarkable durability to persist in specialized rehabilitation agencies.

Ideally, every community should have all of these service delivery models represented in its borders so that rehabilitation programming could be properly individualized. However, even in the largest of American cities, this does not occur. In reality, most blind clients have access to very few service options and especially in small communities, they may be faced with a "take-it-or-leave-it" situation. That is, with only one or two agencies open to them, service is delivered either through them or not at all. Even though a greater number of alternatives exist in larger communities, this does not necessarily guarantee a sufficiently wide range of choices since the agencies in these communities may district their operations or use the same model or approach.

Although philosophical controversy continues to swell around the integration, segregation continuum, the issue is more than academic. The fact is that human life can be shaped differently by these varying approaches. Thus, segregated models tend to stress the development of skills for coping with blindness while integrative models emphasize intergroup socialization and adaptation to unsheltered conditions. Depending upon the type of person he is and upon which type of program he enters, a blind client may emerge as a self-fulfilled individual or as a frustrated person who has been defeated rather than helped by his rehabilitation experience. Rehabilitation is full of zealots who advocate one or another of these approaches. Their arguments constitute resounding summaries of the strengths and weaknesses of all existing models, but with fulsome praise being reserved primarily for the approach of their choice. As in many instances in rehabilitation, this discourse tends to serve the advocates more than they do the target population. The assumption always is that there is a preferred route for all blind (or other handicapped) persons. Current evidence supports another position. This position holds that as many options as possible should be made available to blind persons and those who work with them. The particular option selected by, for, and with a blind individual should be the one that the counselor and client agree holds the greatest promise for him. In this context, pragmatism and a respect for human differences take precedence over dogma and obstinacy.

The implications of this position for the rehabilitation administrator are clear. Whatever the setting, both segregated and integrated experiences are needed by individual blind clients as they progress through their rehabilitation programs. The selection of service components for a blind client should be keyed to client needs rather than professional ideologies. If rehabilitation workers need ego trips to justify some well-established belief they have, other provisions should be made to meet that need. Administratively, the only tenable option in serving blind persons is that of offering a repertoire of services, settings, and facilities so that the most appropriate combination can be selected for each client rather than subjecting him to program rigidities and stereotyping designed to satisfy someone's cherished theories.

Standards for Rehabilitation Programs for the Blind

Whatever the agency setting, rehabilitation programs for blind persons should provide service that is equivalent to, or better than, the basic standard for the field. Accepted standards in this regard have been established by the National Accreditation Council which, after involving a broad sample of leaders and practitioners in various areas of service to blind people, evolved a set of manuals that contain the fundamental requirements for many different types of service to the blind. By and large, these standards represent consensus positions and are reasonable and practical. As time goes by, it is hoped that agencies will generally move well beyond these boundaries into higher levels of performance (as, indeed, a number have already done so). However, administrators who are desirous of measuring their present or proposed rehabilitation programs for the blind against a basic yardstick should use these National Accreditation Council Standards initially for self-study and, hopefully, later on to qualify for NAC accreditation.

National Industries for the Blind, the nationwide coordinating agency for workshops for the blind, maintains a Rehabilitation Services Division which assists associated workshops to work toward the eventual accreditation of their programs. In addition to informing workshops about the values of accreditation and procedures for attaining it, the NIB Rehabilitation Services Division assesses local workshop programs and recommends steps that can be taken to upgrade service and procedures at these facilities. In this connection, administrators should be aware of the Technical Assistance Program of the Rehabilitation Services Administration. In this program, rehabilitation agencies may apply to their respective Regional Rehabilitation Services Administration Offices for support of plans to bring in respected consultants for limited periods of time to evaluate programs (for the blind and other disability groups) and to recommend courses of action designed to upgrade service.

Other Special Administrative Concerns

Funding, managing, and leading a rehabilitation program for blind clients differs little in basic operations from performing similar administrative functions in relation to other disability groups. As indicated earlier, programming does require some special provisions but these are always made in the context of sound general administrative principles and procedures. Yet, there are a few additional administrative variables in which the fact that the clients are blind introduces certain new elements.

Separation from Other Rehabilitation Agencies

Traditionally, rehabilitation programs for the blind have kept themselves aloof from general rehabilitation services. This tendency has been reinforced by the specialized approaches used in this field, the impact of strong differentiated national agencies (such as the American Foundation for the Blind, National Industries for the Blind, and the American Association of Workers for the Blind), the relatively large number of blind persons that are employed in specialized rehabilitation programs, and the seclusive psychology that prevails among workers for the blind which make for certain amount of distrust of outsiders. As a consequence of sequestering itself from the mainstream of American rehabilitation, the field of service to blind persons has not benefited as fully as it should have from sharing in some of the major program and administrative developments that have occurred in the general rehabilitation movement as a whole. Administrators of rehabilitation programs for the blind should consider the advisability of cross-fertilization with other types of rehabilitation programs and the possible adoption of some of the practices that work so well for them in such areas as learning capacities, advocacy, diversified evaluation procedures, openness to change, arranging for specific vocational skill training, and respect for idiosyncratic social and vocational goals.

The Charity Concept

Although most agencies for the blind have moved beyond the point of making blatant appeals to public sympathy and charity, evident residuals of this approach remain in certain locations. Sometimes, the fund-raising exigencies that confront most voluntary organizations induce administrators to compromise with emotional appeals that are used as a means of funding essential agency activities. In other cases, agency executives actually exploit community feelings to maximize public contributions and support. When tempted to exploit the charity route to any degree, rehabilitation administrators should recognize that it is a two-edged sword. While funding possibilities may be enhanced and community interest may be stimulated, this approach simultaneously reinforces concepts of dependency and helplessness. The dilemma is that of reaping all the benefits of emotional appeals with none of the vitiating backlash that deprives blind people of rehabilitation opportunities. One trend is away from extensive reliance on philanthropy and toward more constructive funding by fees, awards, and grants. If this can be done, fewer rehabilitation programs for the blind will be at cross purposes, advocating greater independence for blind persons while concurrently contributing to community conceptions of their dependency.

The Blind Personnel Concept

Suitable employment opportunities for qualified blind professional and clerical workers once were so scarce that job candidates in these occupational categories were forced to seek employment almost exclusively at agencies for the blind. As a matter of conscience, the Boards and the administrators of these specialized programs felt bound to give job preference to the population they were serving. At the same time, they felt a responsibility to set a model for other community employers. It was reasoned that if agencies for the blind failed to hire blind persons, how could they expect others to do so? As time went on, agencies for the blind acquired some exceedingly competent, even brilliant, blind employees as well as a number of less-than-qualified individuals. The issue of preference for blind employment candidates at agencies or programs for the blind has never been fully resolved. However, this much has been decided: whether such preference is given or not, every person hired by such an agency should meet the standards established for his job category. It is now recognized that while providing employment for blind persons is highly desirable, agencies may be defeating their own ends when they take on blind personnel with serious shortcomings who can well damage the lives of many other blind individuals who come to the agency for service.

Summary

Blind clients are different from other rehabilitation clients in a number of specific dimensions. These differences relate to mobility, awareness and control of the environment, communication capabilities, appreciation of the world, cognitive abilities and learning, acceptance in society, opportunities for growth, development, and the burden of being labeled blind. Such differences are so pervasive that they mandate modified rehabilitation programming. Whether such programming is offered in the confines of a general agency or a special agency for the blind, special provisions should be made for different types and qualities of service, including vision rehabilitation, health evaluation and health care, restoration in other sensory and health areas, psychological testing, learning capacities, mental health services, mobility instruction, self-care activities, home responsibilities, communication skills, vocational evaluation and training, and sheltered employment opportunities. Beyond providing for these special needs of blind clients and exercising generally sound administrative judgment and procedures, administrators of rehabilitation programs for blind persons need to take into account the effects of the professional isolation of services for the blind, the widespread concept of charity for blind persons that prevails in the community, and the part that agencies play in prolonging and reinforcing public concepts of the dependency of blind individuals in our society.

REFERENCES

Blank, H. R.: Psychoanalysis and blindness. *Psychoanal Q, 26:*1024, 1957.

Carroll, T. J.: *Blindness.* Boston, Little, Brown, 1961.

Chevigny, H., and Bravenman, S.: *The Adjustment of the Blind.* New Haven, Yale University Press, 1950.

Cholden, Louis S.: *A Psychiatrist Works with Blindness.* New York, American Foundation for the Blind, 1958.

Farrell, G.: *The Story of Blindness.* Cambridge, Harvard University Press, 1956.

Hardy, R. E., and Cull, J. G.: *Social and Rehabilitation Services for the Blind.* Springfield, Thomas, 1972.

Lowenfeld, B.: Psychological foundation of special methods in teaching blind children. In Zahl, P. A. (Ed.): *Blindness.* Princeton, Princeton University Press, 1950.

Lukoff, I., and Whiteman, M.: *The Social Sources of Adjustment to Blindness.* New York, American Foundation for the Blind, undated.

Malikin, D., and Rusalem, H. (Eds.): *Vocational Rehabilitation of the Disabled: An Overview.* New York, New York University Press, 1969.

Richterman, H.: *Guidelines for Rehabilitation Services for Blind Persons.* Unpublished and undated.

Rusalem, H.: *Workshops in the 70's.* New York, National Industries for the Blind, 1968.

Rusalem, H.: *Coping with the Unseen Environment.* New York, Teachers College Press, 1973.

CHAPTER 9

SERVING THE HEARING IMPAIRED AND COMMUNICATIONALLY DISORDERED PERSON IN REHABILITATION FACILITIES

JOAN G. HAMPSON

Introduction

PERHAPS THE MOST SINGULAR attribute which sets the human animal apart from the other creatures with whom we share this planet is our use of language, in the form of speech, as a vehicle for verbal communication. Researchers have demonstrated that bees, ants, dolphins, and probably all mammals possess signaling systems of greater or lesser complexity which approximate simple communicational systems usable for the transmission of relatively concrete messages. Man alone has a language system permitting him to deal with abstract matters and to transmit and preserve his awareness of himself and his world in the form of literature and of history.

In human beings, communications are by no means restricted to verbal behavior. So much has been written about nonverbal communication and body language that such concepts have become a part of the everyday argot of our society. Nonetheless, it remains indisputable that verbal communication is for man the principle avenue for learning and expression, while verbal speech remains the principle vehicle of language and verbal language the primary basis of communication.

One attribute of every undamaged human of whatever race or culture is that he is born with the brain with an innate capacity or substrate for the development of language. Language and speech do not emerge spontaneously, but the capacity to learn a language is an inherent function of the undamaged cerebral substrate.

In the human infant various senses are developed in varying degrees at the time of birth. Vision, for instance, is relatively poorly developed. It has been experimentally established, however, that hearing as well as taste are relatively mature senses even before birth, yet the newborn baby does not have language and speech. It takes fifteen to eighteen months of exposure to sounds of speech before the child is capable of imitating and producing intelligible words, and many more months of exposure and practice before the child has acquired syntactical skills required for stringing words together into meaningful spoken language.

The congenitally hearing-impaired child is deprived of this essential exposure to correct patterns for language modeling. Language for such a child must be acquired by other than the usual sequence of auditory exposure and imitation. It follows, then, that the language and communication problems of an adult, deafened prelingually, are probably greater challenges to the rehabilitation expert than the relatively simple factor of peripheral deafness *per se*. To quote Switzer and Williams (1967), "The communication problem of deaf people overrides and influences all else. It is pervasive, deep and resistant. The deaf person's degree of adjustment and his levels of achievement in every activity relate directly to his skill in communications."

The Nature of Communication

It is axiomatic that a verbal communicational exchange involves a sender and a receiver, who, in turn, produce a message and a response. Reduced to its simplest elements, such an exchange can be thought of schematically as a circular feedback loop.

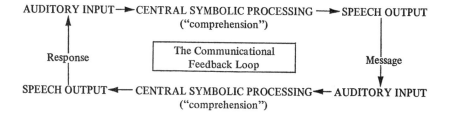

This schema, representing a single verbal exchange between two people, is virtually self-explanatory. The precise nature of what is here labelled central symbolic processing is an immensely complicated neurophysiologic event which, although a matter for a continuing and elegant debate between neurophysiologists and linguistic experts, is beyond the scope of the present chapter. These theoretical constructs, however, have little immediate bearing on the provider of rehabilitation services.

Confronted with a communicationally disordered person seeking rehabilitative assistance, one needs first and foremost to find out where the communicational feedback loop is disrupted. Is the problem one of peripheral hearing, a central processing dysfunction, a speech disorder, or, as would be most usual, some combination thereof?

Types of Hearing Impairment

In attempting to bring some order to the varieties and degrees of hearing-impairment, it is tempting to consider all hearing-impaired persons on one continuum: total deafness to mildly hearing-impaired. But to do so establishes an over-simplification which is liable to do a disservice to many hearing-impaired people. Somewhere along this continuum of impairment there lies a colossal chasm which divides the *deaf* from those called *hard of hearing*, even though the degree of impairment of hearing in some persons classified as hard of hearing may be very severe. It is appropriate, at this point, then, to define these terms.

The definition of *deafness* is at best imprecise in that no iron-clad medicolegal definition exists. One might expect that a reliable test of auditory acuity would be all that would be required. A certain cut-off point would be established, and beyond this limit a person could be considered to be deaf or at another level to be hard of hearing. However, this kind of testing has very little functional utility in differentiating the deaf from the hard of hearing, or in clarifying the degree to which the individual is handicapped. Two individuals with the same degree and patterning of auditory acuity as measured by pure tone thresholds may differ markedly in auditory functioning as measured by speech discrimination tests. Likewise, two individuals with similar auditory functioning as displayed on the audiogram may display grossly divergent sensitivity to sound. *Functional* hearing depends on many factors other than sheer auditory capacity—motivation, age of onset, type of loss, and associated neurological deficits.

So, in the end, the definition of deafness has to be an operational one. The deaf person is one whose hearing loss is so severe that his hearing is not functional for purposes of speech reception, even with amplification. The hard of hearing person is one whose hearing loss varies from very slight to very severe, yet he retains enough hearing that he can depend, with or without amplication, on his ears as his main means of speech reception.

Many deaf children have additional secondary or superimposed disabilities which compound their learning and adjustment problems. For instance, the rubella-damaged infant is frequently additionally compromised; he may have additional neurologic central defects. He may be visually handicapped, or he may have cardiac defects. The Rh-damaged infant may have auditory nerve impairment and, in addition, have generalized brain damage, cerebral palsy, or mental retardation. The list grows longer and the numbers of multi-handicapped deaf rise as medical technology and skills are cutting down birth mortality rates. A damaged infant, who twenty years ago would have not survived, now grows up to be a multiple handicapped adult presenting an enormous challenge to educational, vocational, and rehabilitation specialists.

We do not notice the deaf amongst us as we note the white cane of the blind man or the wheelchair of the paraplegic: the deaf are an invisible minority. Until the final figures of the national census of the deaf becomes available, only estimates of the numbers of deaf and hard of hearing are available. There are roughly five million people in the United States who can be classified as "hearing-impaired," including both deaf and hard of hearing. Of this number, probably 300,000 are deaf by the definition given above. Hard of hearing persons share, to some extent, the problems of deaf persons, and many of them certainly qualify as legitimate candidates for rehabilitative efforts. In general, the hard of hearing person is spared the gross interference with communication through usual channels that is the particular burden of the deaf person and his family.

The Importance of Age at the Time of Onset of the Disability

The chronology of onset of deafness is the single great dividing factor which, in general, determines the degree of disability. Deafness of severe degree from birth, or before language and speech patterns have been established, is by far a greater disadvantage than if the person has had the opportunity, even for a very few childhood years, of experiencing understandable sounds and becoming aware of the symbolic process by which we internalize and organize environmental auditory stimuli into the building blocks of language.

In rehabilitation work with adults in those centers where such services are provided, one is most often dealing with individuals either deaf from birth or deafened prelingually, and who therefore are subject to the greatest degrees of handicap.

Causes of Deafness

Because the etiology of deafness in an individual often has significant bearing on the prognosis and may give clues as to associated handicaps, knowledge of the cause of deafness can be extremely useful for planning the necessary rehabilitation services.

The two major types of hearing loss are (1) conductive losses, which usually result from involvement of the mechanical sound transmitting apparatus of the middle ear, and (2) sensorineural or nerve loss, in which the inner ear structures (i.e. the cochlea) or the auditory nerve and central nerve pathways are affected.

Conductive or Middle Ear Deafness

Conductive or middle ear deafness is most usually caused by infection, i.e. chronic middle ear infections, otitis, and can result in varying degrees of destruction of the middle ear sound-conducting structures. Occasionally, conductive deafness can result from various developmental failures of middle ear structures. Conductive hearing losses are usually of lesser degree than sensorineural losses, but conductive hearing loss is of extreme importance in children living among impoverished conditions in substandard housing and in adverse climates. However, in the population of the United States at large, improved chemotherapy has cut down on conductive hearing losses due to chronic bacterial ear infection. For those conductive losses that still do occur, several microsurgical reconstructive procedures are possible, even when there has been extensive destruction of middle ear structures. Tympanoplasty and other grafting procedures can be done, and artificial prosthetic replacements for the middle ear bony structures are sometimes possible. In favorable cases, considerable restoration of conductive hearing loss is obtained. Medical and surgical interventions in such cases are obviously important rehabilitative measures. It must be noted, though, that physical restoration of hearing does not totally eliminate the disadvantage for the person. Research has shown that when a significant degree of hearing impairment has existed during the early years which are so critical for the development of adequate language skills, the child remains to some degree behind his contemporaries in acquisition of language for years, perhaps indefinitely, even though the surgical result in terms of the audiogram may be superb.

Nerve or Sensorineural Deafness

The secondary major category of deafness is nerve or sensorineural deafness due to inner ear or central causes. Instances of such types of deafness are occurring with probably just as great a frequency as ever among those clients seeking rehabilitation services since the vast majority of hearing impairments fall into the category of sensorineural ones. In most instances, sensorineural deafness occurs early in life or is present at birth, though it may occur in adult life as a result of ototoxic drugs such as the streptomycin group. These days, though, they may be life-saving in certain illnesses which can effectively obliterate the hearing functions of the inner ear. Occasionally, as a result of trauma, tumor, or infection, sensorineural deafness occurs in an adult. There are also a number of conditions, many of a familial-hereditary type, which produce increasing sensorineural deafness beginning in adult years, though not usually progressing to the severe or profound deafness seen in some instances in children.

There are many causes of early profound sensorineural deafness. As a gross approximation, 50 percent of the cases of early profound nerve deafness are hereditarily determined. That is, they are due to genetic causes which are inherited in various ways. Of the 50 percent of cases of early profound deafness that is genetically determined, about 10 percent are transmitted in the dominant mode. The remaining 90 percent of genetic deafness falls into one or another recessive transmission patterns. There are many different genes for recessive deafness, and many different recessively transmitted syndromes associated with deafness exist. If a recessive gene is involved, the child will have inherited an identical recessive gene from each of his parents. If there are 40 or more different recessive genes, the chances of a man and wife having exactly matching recessive genes is remote, though statistically the likelihood is enhanced by intermarriage. Yet, 90 percent of genetic deafness *is* recessive. This clearly points to the extremely wide distribution in the population at large of recessive-type genes for deafness. It is estimated that probably one in every four persons carries a recessive gene for deafness; it is therefore simply random good fortune if we select a mate who does not possess a matching gene. Since the permutations and combinations in genetic possibilities are infinite, it is, of course, perfectly possible for genetically deaf parents to produce only hearing children. It is equally possible for a genetically deaf child to occur in a family where no one can recall any incidence of deafness in any of the forebears for generations. A genetically deaf adult contemplating raising a family should certainly be given the opportunity for expert genetic counseling. Most large university medical centers or teaching hospitals would be able either to provide a medical genetics counseling service or to direct individuals to such a service.

The foregoing discussion has dealt with the 50 percent of early deafness that is genetically determined. We turn now to the other 50 percent of early deafness which may be congenital. Such deafness is present at birth yet *not* genetic: it either results from intrauterine damage to the developing ear structures of the fetus, or it occurs shortly after birth because of Rh damage, lack of oxygen, prematurity, or unascertained causes. Prenatal damage of a non-genetic kind may be due to viral infection of the mother. Although rubella is the most notorious virus in this regard, other viruses can also produce deafness in the fetus. Or, the nongenetic deafness may be due to ototoxic medications given to the mother which cross the placental barrier and damage the vulnerable developing ear structures of the fetus. Rh-antibody incompatibility between the parents has already been referred to, and several kinds of meningitis are notorious deafeners of young children.

It must be added, as a further element of confusion, that some genetic deafnesses are not manifested at birth. Although genetically determined, such hearing loss may not begin until the preschool years or even later.

Sensorineural deafness does not, in general, yield to any medical or surgical techniques that have, as yet, been developed. We cannot wait for the prosthetic developments that may eventually come. We must work with the tools that we have, essentially social and educational, to give the deaf child an opportunity for maximum personal development.

The Importance of Auditory Experiences

The human organism is highly dependent on its senses. Throughout life, but especially in the early days, an individual gathers sensory input and experiences, thus building up bit by bit an awareness of the world and of himself or herself as a unique member of this world. To the deaf infant, and for that matter the deaf adult too, environmental awareness is sharply restricted. Hearing extends our contact with our environment far beyond our line of vision. Our hearing gives us our greatest outreach around us. As normally hearing persons, we can hear in the dark, we can hear around corners, we can, with the right kind of electronic gadgetry, hear around the world. The deaf person who is dependent on the language of sign or of speech reading can hear no further than the horizon of his vision at best. The deaf person cannot hear around corners, nor can he argue in the dark.

For the deaf child, the establishment of effective communication is the central problem issue of his life. Communication, as we have seen, is a two way process involving sender and receiver. As a sender, the deaf person is likely to have deficiencies manifested by inferior language whether signed or spoken. As a receiver, he may read poorly and in his other visual reception, either speech reading or his sign language, his level of understanding may be poor. Whatever educational method has been espoused, oral or manual, he is dependent on visual reception which is a highly artificial substitute, at best, for normal auditory sensory receptive input. In this regard it is noteworthy that the blind child with auditory but no visual clues learns to speak fluently at the normal time, while the child who is profoundly deaf from birth learns to talk, if at all, with agonizing slowness.

The focus on speech development by parents and educators can be too great. It is important that we not confuse speech and language. As important as it is, speech is merely the most usual vehicle of language. Language is the touch-stone of thinking and of reasoning and of communication; communication is perhaps the essence of being human.

The Impact of Hearing Impairment on Personality

The process of personality maturation in any individual is an ongoing learning process which involves conditioning, imprinting, social reinforcement, and all the other experiences that cumulatively determine the emotional, intellectual, and social responses of the individual. In the person profoundly deaf from infancy, the process is identical but the experiences are atypical, distorted, and in some areas completely lacking. Experiences may be different because of the nature of the deficiencies in sensory input, but experiences may also be atypical because of parental response. The degree to which parents can accept the fact of their child's deafness, the degree to which the parents can enrich the child's life both in terms of supportive acceptance and in efforts to compensate for the gaps in the receptive input, will also influence his ultimate personality development.

Without getting involved in specific techniques and details of psychologic testing, it can be said that deaf subjects in formal IQ testing show test results in the same range of IQ test performances as non-deaf subjects. In deaf subjects there are, however, frequently deficiencies in patterns of thinking and reasoning, as well as levels of abstract ability. The deaf persons' tendency to function most adequately at the level of the concrete often conveys a flavor of rigidity to the personality.

There is a commonly held belief that paranoid tendencies and deafness go hand in hand. I think it important to try to dispel that myth. There does not seem to be any good evidence that the incidence of paranoid defenses is any higher among congenitally deaf and pre-lingually deafened persons than in the population at large. However, it is probably a valid observation that there is an excessive degree of suspiciousness and paranoid tendencies in those people who suffer a severe hearing loss *after* growing to maturity as hearing persons.

If there is any valid profile of the personality of the congenitally deaf person, it would have to include general psychologic immaturity, self-centeredness, impulsiveness and low levels of self-esteem. The root cause of all these probably is related to impoverished inner language.

Life Problems of the Hearing Impaired

Interaction with Normal Hearing Persons

Perhaps because of the singularly human attribute of speech and language, hearing people tend to judge a stranger by his speech mannerisms, his vocabulary, his accent and enunciation, in short, his general articulateness. While it is true that in occasional rare instances a profoundly hearing impaired person uses language correctly, speaks with total intelligibility and speech reads (lip-reads) with such skill that "normal" channels of communication with hearing people are available to him, the vast majority of profoundly hearing-impaired people are at a significant disadvantage in communicating with hearing people. For the vast majority of profoundly hearing-impaired people, speech is labored, unnatural sounding, often unattractive, and frequently barely intelligible. Occasionally a profoundly hearing-impaired individual will have available to him no formal communication system of any kind. He must rely, in lieu of spoken language, written language or manual communication (the Language of Signs) upon spontaneous gesture and pantomime.

Inevitably, there is an almost automatic tendency for a hearing person, naive to the problems of deafness, to correlate speech quality and language skills with intelligence and general competence. In point of fact, and documented by much research, the range of intelligence among hearing-impaired persons who have no additional disability falls within the range typical for the population at large.

A small minority of profoundly hearing-impaired people are driven by compulsions of almost neurotic intensity to prove themselves competitive with persons with normal hearing. The fact remains though, that the majority of hearing-impaired people tend to be employed in jobs grossly below their full potential. Unemployment is not typical of the deaf, yet underemployment is virtually the rule. Employers tend to be very wary of non-hearing, non-speaking potential employees. From the point of view of neglect of human resources, underemployment should surely be of major concern. However, and perhaps regrettably, from the point of view of the rehabilitation specialist, unemployment is most usually the focus of attention.

THE TYRANNY OF THE TELEPHONE. Switzer and Williams (1967) have pointed out with great accuracy that "when ears are nonfunctional, the individual's environment shrinks enormously. He is not automatically warned of danger beyond his peripheral vision. The emotional release of beautiful music whether alone or shared with loved ones and friends is not for him. The inspiring speaker at the town hall, the restful chitchat with a seatmate, the effortless absorbing of news and knowledge by word of mouth, by radio, instant sharing in neighborhood excitement, participation in the give and take of the classroom, the awakening telephone call from the desk clerk, deep isolation in a milling crowd, these are a small sample of the thousands and thousands of differences which deprive a deaf person, which require him to adopt uncommon means to compensate." For instance, in contemporary daily living the telephone assumes the characteristics of a tyrant. In the absence of assistance the deaf person with a toothache must either write to or go in person to make an appointment with a dentist. In like manner the dentist would be unable to hire the deaf person even if otherwise qualified to work in his office as a receptionist since telephone skills are an imperative to the smooth functioning of his office. To give further examples is to be redundant. The delight which most of us experience when we can "get away from the telephone" only points up the ubiquitous importance of the telephone in the workaday world.

In contrast to such reality-based limitations, there are myriad pervasive and pernicious ways in which the deaf are discriminated against. Many deaf persons come to be vocationally damaged because, in ways both subtle and obvious, low expectations have been held out for them by others. Almost inevitably they come to have such low expectations of themselves that they eventually become low achievers, functioning much below their innate potential.

Interaction with Other Hearing-Impaired People

> Within the macrocosm of our culture there exists a microcosm made up of deaf people, often referred to as the deaf subculture or the deaf community. The subculture of deaf persons has its roots in their urgent need to nullify the communication barrier. . . . (Williams and Sussman, 1967)

To the uninitiated, the complexity of organizations, the variety of social and recreational opportunities, and other avenues related to civil rights, insurance, and religion, organized by the deaf for the benefit of the deaf community, must necessarily come as a great surprise. Related to this is the fact that deaf persons tend to concentrate geographically in areas where there are other deaf people; this phenomenon facilitates the development of social organizations and marital opportunities. It is reliably estimated that 95 percent of deaf people select deaf marriage partners. The genetic implications of this are obvious.

The point to be made here is that the rehabilitation worker should be aware of an important and extensive deaf subculture wherein he may find many resources upon which he can draw in working with deaf clients.

Rehabilitation Services for Hearing-Impaired and Communicationally Disordered People

If underemployment rather than unemployment is the hallmark of the deaf, then under-service rather than absence of service is characteristic of most rehabilitation services for the deaf.

Adequate, high quality rehabilitative service for the hearing-impaired is extremely expensive; even if cost were of no concern, trained personnel to staff these facilities are in extremely short supply. In the final analysis, however, the expense over the long-term is certainly worthy of attention if only in terms of the tax-dollar return to the community from rehabilitees.

The deaf are a singularly mobile group as compared with many other rehabilitation groups, and no special or extraordinary provision need be made by the facility with respect to accessibility. It stands to reason, though, that there are advantages to having the facility located in an area with access to job-sampling opportunities and with easy provision for follow-up services to rehabilitated clients as they move into independent employment in the community. Nor need there be any concern about the motivation of the hearing-impaired, or their willingness to use the services of the rehabilitation facility once they are established. As a group the deaf are very highly motivated toward acquiring economic self-sufficiency. Despite barriers of hearing and speech, there exists in the deaf community a highly integrated network of communication, and news of the availability of good services will spread quickly; case-finding is not a major problem, as it may be among the blind.

If a rehabilitation facility is going to give adequate service to the profoundly hearing-impaired, there must be a sufficient number of people on the staff of the facility who can communicate with the deaf clients—whether this be in sign language or with the patience to try to understand the sometimes tortured oral efforts of deaf clients to communicate. Communication is the *sine qua non* of adequate rehabilitation services.

In planning for the rehabilitation of the individual client, we can consider two phases. The first would be the evaluative or assessment phase in which the individual's needs are determined; the second phase is an implementation phase in which remedial measures are undertaken as indicated by the evaluation. It is imperative for the success of this approach that the same team responsible for the evaluation is also responsible for implementing their own recommendations. Although I have repeatedly used the term rehabilitation in the foregoing, it may often be more precise to consider it a process of "habilitation," particularly for the prelingually deafened, since many clients, though chronologically adults, will not have had a prior opportunity for the development of independent living skills. Rehabilitation is a team enterprise; no one rehabilitation expert can possibly have the expertise to evaluation all of the specific requirements of the hearing-impaired person. For an ideal evaluation there should be, before the individual is accepted into the facility, a *social work evaluation* and a *general medical evaluation*. When the client arrives at the facility the number one priority, in point of time, is a *comprehensive audiologic assessment,* and when the audiograms have been done, the client should be referred to an otologist. Other facets of the evaluation must include a *speech and communication assessment*, a *psychological evaluation* to explore the individual's inherent intellectual capabilities and potential as well as personality assessment, a *psychiatric evaluation,* a *vocational assessment* to determine interests and aptitudes, an *educational assessment* for appraisal of the individual's present level of academic achievement. Finally, it is highly desirable that the client be in residence at the facility for a period so that the staff may evaluate the client's *everyday living skills.* From the foregoing it will be clear that for the profoundly hearing-impaired clients, it is imperative that each member of the evaluation team be able and willing to communicate in whatever combination of sign and verbal speech best meets the needs and preferences of the client.*

Social Work Evaluation

A good social work evaluation of the hearing-impaired client would not differ substantially from any standard social work intake interview but it should, if possible, be done in the client's home, as this provides an added dimension to the social data. It should include the referral information and something about the expectations of the client and his family as to outcome of the evaluation. It should include something about the etiology of the hearing loss, insofar as it is known, including information about hearing-impairment in other members of the family. A sketch of the client's early-life environment is important as well as other standard social data.

The educational data should be as comprehensive as can be obtained, including data on the types of schools the client attended, i.e. whether the schools were residential schools for the deaf or public schools, with or without special provisions for deaf or hearing-impaired children. Inquiry should be made into the vocational history of the individual and something of his attitudes toward his status as a hearing-impaired person. Behavioral observations would, of course, be relevant, including comments on

* More than five years ago, Clyde E. Mott, M.A., Director of the Seattle Hearing & Speech Center, having long recognized the need for comprehensive rehabilitative services for profoundly hearing-impaired adults, initiated a pilot project from which the present evaluation format has evolved. The author acknowledges with gratitude the opportunity to participate in the growth and development of this program, which at the time of this writing is unique in this country. Members of the present evaluation team, in addition to the author, are: Joseph Afanador, Ph.D. (Coordinator); Bill Boland (Residential Aide Supervisor); Janis K. Collins, M.S.P.A. (Speech Pathologist); Roger M. Falberg, M.A. (Psychologist); Donald G. Harvey, Ph.D. (Audiologist); Allie M. Joiner, B.S. (Vocational Counselor) and Larry L. Petersen, M.A. (Education Specialist). It is of interest that four members of this professional team are themselves deaf. The author is indebted to all members of this evaluation team for providing a challenging and intellectually stimulating opportunity for collaboration.

ease of rapport with the client and family and the quality of communication between the client and his family.

Audiologic Assessment

In some quarters there has been a questioning of the need for audiologic assessment as part of the total appraisal of the profoundly hearing-impaired individual. It is the author's strong conviction that an audiologic evaluation can contribute immeasurably to the total understanding of the present status and potential of the hearing-impaired individual. The deaf person himself may question the necessity for further audiologic examinations. He may need to have explained to him that the audiologic examinations are necessary to enable him to live as fully and up to his potential as possible and that even marginal hearing is important to his environment. His hearing loss must be defined in degree and quality. Hearing strengths and weaknesses must be ascertained; often clients do not know this themselves. In ordinary circumstances, the auditory evaluation will begin with routine air and bone conduction pure-tone testing, and will continue with speech threshold and discrimination testing. The test materials currently available for the audiologic assessment of discrimination in less than profound hearing disabilities does not in general lend itself to this particular type of testing. The audiologist will need to devise test material appropriate to the hearing levels of the individual client.

These examinations should be followed by free-field pure tone and speech testing both aided and unaided. If the client is already a hearing aid user, obviously his function with his own hearing aid would be used with this test. B&K testing, i.e. testing with the Bruel and Kjaer instrumentation, should follow next. This testing is essentially an electroacoustic analysis of the frequency response and distortion characteristics of the particular hearing aid. If testing to this point suggests in any way that the client's auditory performance could be enhanced by an aid other than his present one, a trial of alternate aides should be made. If his performance with an alternate aid seems to offer an advantage, then he would be directed to an appropriate hearing aid dealer for the filling of his hearing aid prescription, and a new hearing aid mold if necessary. Once fitted, B&K rechecking of the new aid should be done to insure that the individual instrument does, in fact, conform to the electroacoustical performance specified and that it is functioning properly. This will supplement the client's personal impression of the instrument. If a new instrument is prescribed, diagnostic therapy should be begun. This is extremely important. At least twice-weekly diagnostic training sessions for a three week period should be begun so that before a final decision for purchase, the audiologist and the client can be fully sure that the hearing aid is the ideal instrument for him. Diagnostic training of this kind will help the individual to function better with the prescribed aid. Diagnostic auditory training may also occasionally be indicated for the long-term hearing aid user whose own aid is determined to be optimal for his needs.

Impedance-Bridge testing may be indicated. This type of test determines the conductive competence of the middle ear. In profoundly hearing-impaired individuals, the standard bone conduction tests are not adequate to show small but significant air-bone gaps, yet the determination of the existence of such additional conductive impairment may be of immense importance and may indicate if medical or surgical intervention is possible.

At some point in the audiologic evaluation, a referral must be made to an otologist who should specifically state as a result of his examinations that the client is or is not suited for wearing a hearing aid in either or both ears. It is the otologist's responsibility to establish that there are no medical contraindications to hearing aid usage. Many otologists feel that they are at an advantage if their examination can be performed when the results of preliminary audiologic examinations are available to them, since the audiologist may have access to more sophisticated tests than are available in the otologist's office.

In many forms of hearing-impairment there is some degree of interference with vestibular function, so that the client may complain of problems of balance and dizziness. Indeed, in some mildly hearing-impaired persons this is the major subjective complaint, and may in fact be disabling in its degree. The otologist may be in a position to ameliorate these complaints by medical means. In certain circumstances electrocochlear testing or electronystagmography can provide critical data.

If it is established that the client can benefit from the fitting of a hearing aid, aural rehabilitation should be commenced. This should be geared to the special auditory difficulties that can be overcome by trained use of the hearing aid. It should be emphasized that many profoundly hearing-impaired people have very strongly set attitudes about hearing aid use and may be misinformed and apprehensive that the goal of fitting a hearing aid is to convert them into oral people capable of speech. Each client must be reassured that the objective of fitting him with an optimal hearing aid is to give him the maximum potential that he himself can use efficiently. Not all people, even with the most minimal residual hearing, are able to profit from hearing aid use. In some, the range between the comfort level and the maximum gain for effectiveness of the instrument is so small that it simply isn't practical for the person to use an electronic aid. In occasional instances the audiologist may even recommend that the hearing aid user give up the use of an aid, since it may be judged to affect his vocational or general social performance. Despite these limitations, however, it is important to fit and give a trial of training in the case of marginal hearing aid users. One simply cannot tell by study of the audiograms alone which clients may profit substantially from the use of the hearing aid. Paramount in these decisions is the patient's attitude. In no case should the audiologist go against the wishes and biases of the individual toward hearing aid use.

Speech and Communication Assessment

In the communication assessment of the moderately hearing-impaired individual, the client's capacity to communicate is evaluated in three dimensions: 1) his communication by writing, 2) his communication by speech, and 3) his communication by the Language of Signs, or Manual English. In each of these areas the client is evaluated in terms of both his receptive and expressive abilities. For the profoundly hearing-impaired population there is a relative scarcity of formal test material and the speech clinician may need to use considerable ingenuity in modifying existing tests or devising new ones. In testing for receptive communication ability a written form of the Peabody Picture Vocabulary test is used. This needs to be keyed to the reading ability of the individual. A test of ability to follow written directions is also used. As a typical test item, the individual may be requested in writing to "cross out the last 't' in every word." At a somewhat more sophisticated level the Gochnour Idiom Test is useful to evaluate the individual's capacity for idiomatic usage. Common expressions such as "goof off" and "drop out" are typical examples.

Of standard tests, the auditory perception subtest of the I.T.P.A. (Illinois Test of Psycholinguistic Abilities) is useful. This is normally administered verbally, but it is given in written form to profoundly hearing-impaired subjects. This test progresses from very simple single word and two-word combinations to increasingly abstract phrases.

The receptive portion of the Northwestern Syntax Screening Test is also used. Again, this is normally given verbally but is administered in written form for the profoundly hearing-impaired person. This tests knowledge of parts of speech and grammatical and syntactical competence.

For the receptive portion of the evaluation of the understanding of speech there are no formal tests at the primitive level. The examiner begins by asking loosely structured questions such as "how old are you?" and "where do you live?" All are obvious biographical questions which the subject will expect to be asked. The test will proceed to test the understanding of somewhat more abstract words and carrier phrases such as "put the key under the box." If the subject's performance is superior up to this point, the examination may proceed to more formal testing such as the Peabody Picture Vocabulary Test, this time administered verbally.

Speech reading skills may also be tested formally. The Utley Speech Reading Test may be administered both aided and unaided by amplification. Some examiners use unvoiced speech, though most commonly the examination is done in voiced speech unaccompanied by sign or gesture.

If it is deemed necessary, speech reading skills can be tested in full face, three quarter profile and full profile. The importance to the client of these tests is open to debate. In virtually every situation where the hearing-impaired client relies heavily upon speech reading, he would be careful to insure a face-to-face orientation.

Receptive ability in manual communication would be determined by finger spelling or signing very simple words, progressing to more complicated phrases and asking the subject to write down what has been communicated.

Expressive Abilities: The expressive tests of communication skills include asking the subject to write a paragraph using key words such as "old," "does," "area." The sentences produced are analyzed for complexity, accuracy of syntax, linguistic structure, and richness of vocabulary.

Formal psychologic testing materials for the profoundly hearing-impaired subjects are scarce. Though considered relatively obsolescent by contemporary workers, the Picture Story Language Test may be useful to those with no other testing tools available.

At a more formal level for expressive language two subtests of the ITPA may be used: (1) the Grammatic Closure Test presented in the form of written stimuli, and (2) the Auditory Association Test, which in essence tests the ability of the individual to understand the predictabilities of English, i.e. "Snow is white; grass is . . . . . ."

Another test often used is the Engelmann Basic Concept Inventory, again, presented in written form.

The majority of the foregoing tests were originally designed for use with normally or mildly hearing-impaired children. It should be understood, therefore, that in their use with profoundly hearing-impaired adults, the results should be interpreted in terms of relative functional ability rather than strictly by the age norms set up for the tests as originally designed.

As a final aspect of the examination of the expressive modalities of speech and language, there should be an examination to insure intactness of the peripheral speech mechanisms. Does the palate move appropriately during phonation attempts? Does the tongue have full freedom of movement in every direction?

The voice quality must be evaluated. Is the speech controlled and appropriate? What of the quality of the voice? Is the individual able to monitor his own vocal productions for optimal volume? How appropriate is his inflection, intonation and cadence? Occlusion, dental and other factors which may influence articulation should also be appraised.

Articulation tests in profoundly hearing-impaired subjects of necessity must be more informal than formal. A subject is asked to construct sentences and a speech sample is obtained which is later analyzed phonetically. If speech is relatively well developed, the Expressive portion of the Northwest Syntax Screening Test may be used. A recorded sample of speech may be transcribed and analyzed for articulatory defects, but this is an extremely cumbersome and time-consuming test and may be unnecessary for most purposes.

With regard to the third dimension of communication assessment, that of communication in the Language of Signs, it is of course necessary that the examiner be familiar with manual langauge if the test is to be feasible. Again, using informal rather than formal tests, an appraisal is made of the client's ability to use signs both expressively and receptively.

Psychological Evaluation

Many standard psychological tests have been found to be feasible to administer to profoundly hearing-impaired subjects and to yield reliable and useful information and data for use by the rehabilitation team:

Intellectual Functioning

1. Wechsler Adult Intelligence Scale (WAIS) for subjects sixteen years of age and up
2. Wechsler Intelligence Scale for Children (WISC) for subjects under sixteen years of age

While it may seem almost axiomatic that the Verbal section of the WAIS and WISC would be inappropriate for the profoundly hearing-impaired individual, it has been demonstrated that a psychologist skilled in communicating with the hearing-impaired can indeed administer the verbal test and can thereby glean a great deal of useful information that would otherwise be unavailable. It stands to reason, however, that the scores attained on the verbal subtests would not be included in the calculation of the total IQ score.

In subjects whose performance on the WAIS is extremely marginal, the following tests may sometimes produce useful data:

3. Arthur Points Scale of Performance, Test II, 1946 revision
4. Arthur Adaptation of the Leiter International Performance Scale
5. S.R.A. Nonverbal Form H (Science Research Associates) is an excellent measure of nonverbal concept formation.

Projective Tests

Projective tests to assess personality characteristics, though lacking, some feel, in reliability and validity, can be given to deaf clients. Many studies now indicate that such tests, used indiscriminately, have little value in making accurate predictions about behavior. In the hands of a skilled psychologist, however, who takes into account the total social and behavioral history of the individual, such tests can play a part in understanding a client's psychological characteristics. Three such tests in common use with profoundly hearing-impaired clients are (1) Draw-a-Person Test, (2) Thematic Apperception Test (T.A.T.), and (3) Make-a-Picture Story (M.A.P.S.) for children and teenagers. It is only the most exceptional hearing-impaired subject who has the language skills and knowledge of idiom to warrant use of the well known MMPI.

Memory Perception and Perceptuomotor Performance Tests

Tests of memory perception and perceptuomotor performance are of extreme importance in the evaluation of hearing-impaired subjects since there is a high association between disturbed performance in these areas and hearing-impairment when the etiology of the hearing loss is due to prenatal viral infection or perinatal damage such as Rh-incompatibility or anoxia. Indeed, it is sometimes the findings obtainable from these tests of memory and perception that provide the most significant clue to the coexistence of a central language disorder or subtle degrees of generalized organic cerebral damage. Tests usually used include the Bender Visual-Motor Gestalt, the Graham-Kendall Test, and the Weigel-Goldstein-Scheerer tests of Abstract and Concrete Thinking.

The Psychiatric Evaluation

The psychiatrist brings to the evaluation of the deaf client the benefit of a medical background and training, plus specific training in psychological medicine and behavioral science. The psychiatrist should have a working knowledge of the Language of Signs. With this exception, psychiatric evaluation of the hearing-impaired individual requires only those basic skills and interviewing techniques required for any good psychiatric assessment. The psychiatrist should be prepared, however, to spend three or four times as long evaluating the profoundly hearing-impaired person than would normally be spent with the average hearing person.

The psychiatrist's examination of the client should review the usual areas of personality functioning, including a mental status examination. The psychiatrist should also talk with any other physicians involved in the client's total care so as to become aware of related medical problems either past or current. By virtue of his or her training, the psychiatrist will be attuned to the vast amount of information that one can get by careful observation of nonverbal behavior.

The psychiatrist's training as a physician will be called upon with surprising frequency in the supervision of associated general medical problems and in the assessment of physical problems which may be present in addition to the deafness, e.g. deafness associated with cerebral palsy, encephalitis, or epilepsy.

In the more traditional psychiatric sense, the psychiatrist will also investigate those factors of family and social background that may be relevant to the client's present or future adjustment. In assessing the client's present life situation, many factors will be considered: with whom and in what style the client lives; what the client's work and educational experiences may have been; what the client may see as his goals for the future and the realism of these goals. The client's friendships and relationships with the opposite sex will be inquired about, as well as his hobbies and recreational interests. Since religion often plays an important role in the life of the profoundly hearing-impaired, it too should be noted. The client's experience with alcohol and drugs should be explored. Although sometimes considerable ingenuity will be needed, the object of the initial evaluation will be to get as comprehensive a picture as possible of the client's ego strengths, self-concepts, and general social competence. If formal psychotherapy is indicated as a result of the initial appraisal, the psychiatrist should be prepared to work psychotherapeutically with the client.

If the client is a hearing aid user, his attitude toward the use of the aid should be explored by the psychiatrist as well as by the audiologist. Surprisingly, it will often be found that a different version will be given to the psychiatrist. The psychiatrist may find, for example, that the client had sought to ingratiate himself with the audiologist by demonstrating enthusiasm for a hearing aid when in fact his true feelings indicate ambivalence or disdain.

In many instances, medication for emotional disturbance is clearly indicated; the psychiatrist is the logical person to assume responsibility for the management of this type of pharmacotherapy.

Educational Evaluation

The purpose of educational testing is to establish the level of academic achievement in basic vocabulary skills, reading skills, receptive and expressive written language and mathematical-computational skills. The standard tests that are used are

1. Gates Basic Vocabulary Reading Test
2. California Achievement Test (Form W), Norms 1963
   a. Reading subtest

   b. Arithmetic-math subtest

   c. Language (receptive) subtest

3. Written Composition Test. In this, the examiner shows the subject a specific standard picture and asks the subject to write a composition about the picture. The productions vary from a simple listing or naming of objects in the picture to richly embellished stories several paragraphs long. The compositions are analyzed with reference to expected norms derived from experience with clients from various educational backgrounds, prelingually and post-lingually deafened, and with varying degrees of hearing impairment and possible additional handicaps.*

Vocational Evaluation

The full vocational evaluation is undeniably time-consuming. Fortunately certain of the tests can be satisfactorily administered to clients in small groups. All of the tests are standard, published instruments. The following test battery has been found to be adequately comprehensive:

I. Interest

   A. Weingarten's Picture Interest Inventory

   B. Vocational Exploratory Picture Inventory (experimental)

   C. Occupational Interest Inventory

      1. Intermediate—Low Verbal Clients

      2. Advanced—High Verbal Clients

   D. Strong Vocational Blank for Men (for Women)—Given only to High Verbal Clients

   E. Minnesota Vocational Interest Inventory—Given only to High Verbal Clients

II. Aptitude

   A. Revised Minnesota Paper Form Board Test

   B. Minnesota Clerical Test

III. Dexterity

   A. Crawford Small Parts Dexterity Test (two tasks)

---

* For normative data for this important test, the interested professional may contact the developer of the test, Larry L. Petersen, M.A., Education Specialist, c/o Seattle Hearing and Speech Center, 18th and Madison, Seattle, Washington.

    B. Purdue Pegboard (four tasks)

    C. Stromberg Gross Movement Dexterity Test (two tasks)

    D. Bennet's Hand-Tool Dexterity Test

IV. Supplementary Tests—contingent on interest and aptitude testing

    A. The Meier Art Tests

        1. Art Judgment

        2. Aesthetic Perception

    B. Mechanical Comprehension Test (Paper-and-Pencil Task)

    C. Flanagan Industrial Tests

        1. Assembly

        2. Electronics

        3. Judgment and Comprehension

        4. Mathematics and Reasoning

        5. Precision

    D. Typing Test for Business

    E. Tower Systems Tests

        1. Clerical (ten series)

        2. Drafting (five series)

        3. Mail Clerk (one out of ten series)

        4. Optical Mechanics (one out of ten series)

Everyday Living Skills

The final dimension of evaluation is of great importance in understanding a client's abilities and limitations in a wide range of aspects of daily living. There is no formal protocol of tests that can be spelled out here, but vitally important data can be obtained by observation of the client in the course of daily living. Such skills as food-buying, menu planning, cooking, personal grooming, money management, use of recreation time as well as more subtle observations on peer-group relations, and willingness to accept supervision and direction comprise the basis for the evaluation of everyday living skills.

The foregoing outline represents the vital elements of an evaluation of a deaf client. Lengthy though this evaluation may seem and although there are minor areas of overlap, each facet of the evaluation adds its unique contribution to a three dimensional picture of the client. There are no true redundancies.

For many multi-handicapped clients, additional examinations and treatment by specialists in internal medicine, ophthalmology, physical medicine, neurology and other medical specialties, or by dentists, occupational therapists or physiotherapists will be indicated. Family planning services should be made available.

It is clear that the complete comprehensive evaluation outlined here will not be necessary for the evaluation and treatment of every hearing-impaired client. For instance, in the case of a moderate, adventitious hearing loss in a mature individual where speech and language are fully developed, the only service required might be an audiologic examination, otologic examination, and the fitting of an appropriate hearing aid with auditory training in maximizing its usefulness. But, for the profoundly hearing-impaired person, particularly one congenitally or prelingually deafened, no component of the evaluation is dispensible.

Interpreting Services—Another Essential

When in the course of evaluating or training, the deaf person is obliged to interact with a hearing person unversed in sign language, the presence of an interpreter is essential. Written exchanges are time consuming and cumbersome at best, and the deaf person, because of language deficiencies, will most likely not to be able to express himself fully in clear and understandable written form. There exists a national organization of well-trained interpreters for the deaf who have been tested and certified by the National Registry of Interpreters for the Deaf, Inc.* Most large urban areas will have a cadre of such individuals. The organization was still in its infancy at the time of this writing and the rehabilitation specialist may need to be resourceful in locating a qualified interpreter. The "Language Bank" listing under "Translators and Interpreters" in the Yellow Pages of the telephone book may help in locating qualified assistance.

Some states have enacted legislation which mandates the presence of a qualified interpreter for every deaf person involved in a legal proceeding. Interpreting is a professional skill for which a local fee schedule has usually been established. The re-

---

* P. O. Box 1339, Washington, D.C. 20013.

habilitation specialist should be prepared to allocate sufficient funds for the provision of this essential rehabilitation service.

Training, Remediation and Therapy

At the conclusion of the evaluation, a meeting which includes all members of the evaluation team, with an interpreter if necessary, must generate a rehabilitation plan tailored to the needs of the individual. Occasionally the remedial plan will be one that can be implemented in a matter of weeks; more usually the various aspects of training and treatment will continue concurrently for months and in some instances years.

Even a cursory discussion of the many modalities of training, remediation and treatment would go far beyond the space alloted to this chapter. Each professional on the evaluation team will bring with him abundant expertise from his professional background to carry out his particular therapeutic task.

Also, it is obvious that there are a host of speech and communication disorders which fall into categories quite apart from those associated with hearing-impairment. Post-stroke aphasias, post-laryngectomy patients, speech dysfluencies such as stuttering and articulation disorders are a few examples. Again, it is beyond the dimensions of this chapter to deal with these special problems.

Conclusion

It must be reiterated that the effective rehabilitation of the profoundly hearing-impaired person is often time consuming and expensive. The question could be asked "can it be afforded?" Expensive though it is, the question should be asked "can it not be afforded?" From the purely cost/benefit point of view the answer is clear. A recent study in the state of Washington showed that for every one dollar of tax money spent on rehabilitation of *all* disabilities, the average anticipated lifetime tax dollar return to the community is eleven dollars per person. For every one dollar of tax money spent on the rehabilitation of the hearing-impaired, the tax return to the community is projected to be $26.20 per person!

The whole thrust of rehabilitation efforts for deaf persons

should be directed not to speech skills, not to specific auditory improvement, not even to language skills *per se* but to providing whatever it takes to insure that the deaf person comes to be someone who can function as a self-confident, responsible, productive human being, using his innate potential to the maximum and requiring minimal special consideration from society.

REFERENCES

Switzer, M. E., and Williams, B. R.: Life problems of deaf people. *Arch Environ Health, 15:*249-256, 1967.

Williams, B. R., and Sussman, A. E.: Social and psychological problems of the deaf. In *Counseling with Deaf People,* New York, N.Y.U. School of Education, 1971.

SUGGESTED FURTHER READING

Eisenson, J.: *Adult Aphasia.* New York, Appleton-Century-Crofts, 1973.

Mindel, E. D., and Vernon, M.: *They Grow in Silence.* Silver Spring, National Association of the Deaf, 1971.

Schlesinger, H. S., and Meadow, K. P.: *Sound and Sign.* Berkeley, University of California, 1971.

Stuckless, E. R. (Ed.): *Behavioral Aspects of Deafness.* Proceedings of National Research Conference on Behavioral Aspects of Deafness. Washington, D. C., U. S. Department of Health, Education, and Welfare, 1965.

Chapter 10

SERVICES FOR DISABLED YOUTH FROM PUBLIC SCHOOL PROGRAMS

Robert Mather and James E. Trela

IN OUR DEMOCRATIC industrial society where an informed citizenry and skilled labor force are thought to be essential national strengths, the public schools are charged with the responsibility for educating *all* youth to the maximum of their individual abilities. One important approach views education as an investment by both society and the individual. From its educational investments society receives a labor force with a high level of technical skill, competence, and productivity which in turn makes continued economic development and growth possible. The individual from his or her investment receives increased earnings made possible by the acquisition of skill and competence during the educational process (Pavalko, 1968). Not all students, however, are able to profit fully from the standard educational curriculum. The result is the loss of human resources and the continued existence of individuals who are in varying degrees dependent and separated from society's social and economic structures. Because of the inabilities of general education to appropriately meet the educational needs of young people with various impairments, special education programs have been developed. The purpose of this chapter is to identify how the broad range of rehabilitation services can be extended and how the rehabilitation facility can provide an effective transitional link to the world of work for disabled students.

Background

Special education here refers to programs which are especially designed to meet the needs of the disabled. To identify, within a specific setting, the types of disabilities for which special education programs have been developed, the Cleveland Board of Education's 1972-1973 student population was examined. Out of approximately 137,000 students attending Cleveland schools, 9,320 were enrolled in special education classes. The largest group of special education students (4,825) was speech impaired and received special speech therapy. The second largest group (3,621) was the Educable Mentally Retarded (EMR). The remainder of the disabled youth fell into the following areas: deaf, 196; hard of hearing, 30; partially seeing, 111; crippled, 241; seriously emotionally disturbed, 32; blind 44, and learning disabled, 220.

Some of the special education programs developed for disabled youth take the form of work study programs which attempt to facilitate the transition from school to work and from the student role to the worker role, to teach the social norms governing the work role, and to inculcate the attitudes and skills essential to competitive employment. Schools have used a variety of approaches to provide initial work experience for disabled youth in work-study programs. A thorough examination of this approach is presented by Kolstoe and Frey (1965). One approach is the assignment of students to work stations within the school involving such tasks as messenger, clerical and maintenance work. A second approach has been the use of work samples from industry in the school setting. Other special education programs have brought together the school and community to provide a comprehensive program for disabled youth. Hence, a third approach has emphasized the assignment of students to work stations within the business and industrial community. The goal, of course, is to bring the student in contact with "real-life" work situations. Finally, a fourth approach has emphasized the utilization of rehabilitation facilities to provide work experiences and supportive services. Legislation in some states now makes it possible for schools to arrange for services from established rehabilitation facilities that have a contract workshop phase.* This approach most nearly makes the transition to the world of work and distinguishes between the student and work roles. Under this law it is possible for students to spend part of their school time in rehabilitation facilities for work experience and the rest of their time in classroom study geared to vocational information and vocationally oriented academic subjects.

For the purposes of identification, the youthful disabled from public schools that are served in rehabilitation facilities will primarily be sixteen to nineteen years old, in grades 9 through 12, and have identifiable learning problems and disabling vocational handicaps. With the educable mentally retarded (EMR) representing the most likely group to participate in a rehabilitation facility, this chapter will primarily focus on the EMR's needs and problems. This group includes individuals with an IQ range between fifty and eighty. However, it is important to add that in addition to mental retardation, many students have secondary disabilities. For example, the study of a work experience program conducted at Vocational Guidance and Rehabilitation Services in Cleveland, Ohio found that approximately half of the students had secondary disabilities in addition to mental retardation (O'Toole and Mather, 1971). The secondary conditions included vision and hearing disabilities, weight problems, social-emotional disorders, and neuromuscular difficulties. Smaller numbers were handicapped by endocrine, respiratory, cardiovascular or convulsive disorders. Also, the majority of the above students came from socially disadvantaged areas of the inner-city, which further handicapped them in attempting to compete in the job market. Hence, many of the school's disabled youth are handicapped by physical and psychological disorders and may be socially disadvantaged in addition to being mentally re-

---

* In some instances schools have established sheltered work programs and operated their own workshop. An example is the Kent County Michigan Program which established and operated a subcontract work program. Students spent one-half-day in the workshop and the other half-day in the study program, thus getting a balance between work and study. See F. G. Warren, "Kent County Occupational and Educational Training Project, Progress Report" (unpublished, 1963).

tarded. All of these problems then must be dealt with in the rehabilitation process.

This chapter focuses on (1) the nature and effectiveness of work-study programs for disabled youth, (2) planning for a work-study program, (3) facility services, and (4) the organizational problems that may attend the development of such a program.

Facility-Based Work-Study Programs

The intent of this section is to describe the role of a community rehabilitation facility, separate from the public schools, in training vocationally disabled youth to enter the labor market on a competitive basis. Inasmuch as the transition from school to work has been a difficult one for those with impairments, the need to provide work experiences to the youthful disabled prior to completing public school has long been apparent. A program involving work experiences in combination with basic educational experiences was indicated when disabled clients were referred to rehabilitation facilities three to five years *after* they had dropped out of or completed special education classes. It has been felt that a preventive program designed to train youthful disabled students in good work attitudes and behavior could prepare them for entry into the labor market as acceptable employees.

Many states have various levels of work-study programs. Typically, as in Ohio, many of the school systems have a four level approach. Each of the levels seeks to further develop work skills and functional attitudes toward work, and facilitate the transition from school to the world of work.

The work-study I level program emphasizes occupational orientation. Classroom instruction involves the student in an exploration of many occupational areas. Specific occupational areas can be selected on the basis of student interest, availability in the community, or through the use of resources such as the *Dictionary of Occupational Titles,* the *Occupational Outlook Handbook,* and the *Occupational Survey.* The purpose of this instruction is to increase the student's knowledge and awareness of the world of work by examining many occupations and answering the following questions about each: What skills are required for the job? What training and experience is required for the job? What is the future demand for workers? and How does one obtain employment in the job?

Classroom instruction can be effectively supplemented by having resource people from the community come to the classroom or through field trips to local industries. Finally, short fifteen minute periods of in-school work experiences can provide the student with an opportunity to explore work situations requiring different skills. This process, in turn, provides data for further teacher instructional planning and may be the first step toward creating work expectations in the student which are consistent with aptitude and ability.

The work-study II level program emphasizes the development of a vocational plan. First, more detailed information on jobs is provided. Also, longer periods of planned work experiences in school laboratory settings provide the students with an opportunity to actually develop particular work skills. Information gained through these experiences, combined with scores on interest inventories and aptitude tests, provides teachers with further vocational planning material.

In work-study III level programs the major emphasis is on helping the student implement his vocational plan. For some students this may mean more specific instruction or training within the schools, but for many, implementation of the vocational plan may involve the community rehabilitation facility. Training at a rehabilitation facility may consist of between one and three hours a day when school is in session. This level is usually for the 9th, 10th, and 11th grade students ranging in ages from sixteen through eighteen years. The type of experiences provided in a rehabilitation facility at this point emphasizes vocational assessment or work evaluation. This gives students half-day experiences on standardized work samples and other tasks which allow for situational evaluation. These work samples should represent the kinds of tasks performed by workers in local industry. The work samples are usually time studied and based on normal expectations for non-handicapped workers.

The students are timed on each sample and their rates are compared to normal worker rates. This information becomes the basis for their work experiences in the rehabilitation facility. A more detailed description of the work evaluation process will be attempted later.

The work-study IV level is the final phase in the developmental sequence of preparing students for the adult world-of-work. The major objective is again to help the student implement his vocational plan by facilitating the transition from school to employment. It has been found that many students need to experience full-time work for at least part of their senior year. Level IV has as its final goal the successful transition from school to some type of employment, whether it be sheltered or competitive. Students are expected to make a smooth transition from the school work-study program to full-time employment in the community as an adult. Work experience, in many instances, is provided by a rehabilitation facility under the program names of work adjustment, work experience, pre-vocational and adjustment training, personal adjustment training, and worker skill training. Probably the most acceptable and most understood term is work adjustment, and this approach will be discussed in detail later in the chapter.

A number of follow-up studies of former public school EMR's have been made. This considerable volume of research indicates that disabled youth have an improved opportunity for adult success when they have participated in a comprehensive program combining academic preparation and rehabilitation facility work-study experience. These studies and others in a variety of communities over the period of three decades (Baller, 1936; Thomas, 1943; Charles, 1953; Bobroff, 1956; Beekman, 1963; and McFall, 1966) present several consistent and interesting findings. Most important, it has been demonstrated in economic terms that rehabilitation of the EMR is justified. No studies surveyed present evidence of EMR's being incapable of productive work. Certain dated writings of the fifties and sixties (*cf.*, Bobroff, 1956) suggest that given a continuation of wage trends, it appears that young EMR's with a work life of thirty years may be expected to earn about $100,000. A successfully placed EMR has been found to return from $7.00 to $10.00 for every dollar spent on his rehabilitation (Presidents' Committee on Employment of the Handicapped, 1962).

The evidence indicates that the majority of EMR's in the community will be found to be functioning adults earning modest wages in semiskilled or unskilled jobs. A comprehensive study by Jones and Dyck (1969) on work-study program effectiveness documents the employment history of work-study graduates as contrasted with nongraduates. Work-study graduates had a significantly higher employment level (68%) than the total EMR sample (57%), or the work-study dropouts (45%). Work-study graduates also reported significantly higher wages than others ($105 as compared with $94). It may be noted, however, that the employment level for EMR's in general was lower at the time of the study than it was right after leaving school. Even this unfortunate fact, nevertheless, supports the effectiveness of work-study programs. The work-study graduates reported the least decline in employment. Work-study graduates were more likely (than other subgroups) to improve their employment status when present employment, previous employment, and the first job after leaving high school are compared. Not surprisingly, students from special education and work-study programs reported higher wages on their first job after leaving high school than those EMR students who had been in a regular program. Further, work-study graduates appeared to be more reliable employees from the standpoint of tenure. While about 18 percent of the total EMR sample had held the same job since leaving high school, 32 percent of the work-study graduates had remained on the same job. Finally, work-study graduates, as contrasted with dropouts, perceived themselves in a more positive manner with respect to variables such as promptness, taking the initiative, and remaining flexible upon placement in new assignments.

Other research is essentially consistent with the above findings. Approaching the problem from a different perspective, Phelps (1958) notes that there has been very little improvement in the occupational status of EMR's and that the *status quo* has been kept only by those graduating from work-study programs. Continuing work-study programs help the EMR's to secure jobs and maintain their employment longer.* In general, compared to other EMR's, work-study graduates enjoyed a higher employment level, higher wages, lower employment attrition, and greater tenure. They were also more likely to improve their occupational status when they did leave a job, were more financially independent, seemed to be better adjusted economically, enjoyed better home conditions, and, not surprisingly, they had a more favorable attitude toward special education programs. It is clear, then, that full utilization of the services of a rehabilitation facility can have a beneficial impact on EMR's from the local public schools.

Planning and Preparation for a Work-Study Program

The most effective work-study programs are those which anticipate the need for close school-facility cooperation and community involvement. Preparing disabled youth for adult roles and facilitating the transition from school to work is a task that must be shared. Work-study must be conceived as a phase of the total educational process and the school and community rehabilitation facility must assume the following responsibilities:

1. Systematic identification of the disabled youth and their needs.
2. Identification of goals and expected outcomes.
3. Development of a division of labor and specification of the roles of the school, the student, and rehabilitation facility.
4. Establishment of formal cooperative arrangements and patterns of communication.
5. Establishment of standards to insure that the work done by

---

* In spite of such encouraging findings, it appears that those supervising or coordinating work-study programs have met only part of the challenge of their task. They have been successful in improving the employment potential of the work-study graduates but they have not been able to place them in more highly skilled jobs than those who have not graduated from work-study programs. Such students are placed in jobs virtually the same as the jobs that EMR's are securing without work-study programs.

students is of a useful, worthwhile nature and that federal, state and local laws and regulations are met.

6. Assignment of qualified personnel to direct and coordinate the rehabilitation work experience and the instructional program of the school.

7. Development of a course of study and work experience that enables the student to fulfill necessary requirements for graduation.

8. Evaluation of the effectiveness of the cooperative program in terms of its goals and expected outcomes.

Assuming that a need for a work-study program has been established, there is no single formula for successfully initiating a cooperative program between a public school and a rehabilitation facility. A highly recommended beginning, however, should be to organize an advisory committee of individuals representing the organizations which agree to participate in the work-study project. The committee may consist of the director of the rehabilitation facility or the facility administrator responsible for the program, representatives of the state rehabilitation agency, administrators and teachers from the school, interested local businessmen and women, and other community leaders. The purpose of this advisory group is to:

1. suggest approaches to work-study that will effectively utilize existing resources;

2. act as a vehicle for involving various segments of the community and securing the cooperation of each;

3. help disseminate information to interested publics;

4. develop program guidelines and articulate expected outcomes, and

5. help secure funding for the program.

Funding sources appear to be the biggest obstacle in beginning a work-study program. Nevertheless, possibilities for funding include Federal Manpower programs, Department of Health, Education and Welfare grants, State Department of Vocational Education programs, State Bureau of Vocational Rehabilitation programs, and State Department of Mental Health and Hygiene programs to name a few.

Following a commitment of funding for a work-study program the facility, being the provider of services, will usually assume responsibility for orientating relevant others with regard to the dimensions of the program. This should include (1) school administrators, teachers, and non-teachers; (2) students, and their parents; (3) the rehabilitation facility's Board of Directors, administrators, counselors, workshop supervisors, work evaluators, and other supportive staff, and (4) other cooperating and interested public agencies, such as the Board of Mental Retardation, Bureau of Vocational Rehabilitation, Welfare Department, Bureau of Employment Services, and other state and federal offices dealing with youthful disabled students.

An effective way to accomplish this orientation is through an open house at the facility. The distribution of descriptive or written material, slides, and visual inspection of the facility can be an effective means of introducing the program. Questions regarding time schedules, kinds of work, wages, travel, hours, purposes of work evaluation and work adjustment, and future employment should be anticipated. Also, questions about the disposition of discipline problems and school dropouts, basic entrance requirements and performance expectations, and such things as smoking policies, lunch and other work breaks may also be appropriate to the discussion.

Most important, to insure an effective work-study program, the rehabilitation facility must work closely with the state rehabilitation agency, the school, and the student and his family. These liaison and orienting activities must be accomplished, at least in part, before direct services can be rendered to the student.

Liaison with the State Agency

Many of the youths participating in a facility-based work-study program may be eligible for the services of the State Vocational Rehabilitation Agency, the bureau, department or division of Vocational Rehabilitation. For ease of identification, the state agency will be referred to here as BVR. For the student to be eligible for BVR services, he must (1) have a diagnosable physical or mental disability; (2) the disability must be a vocational handicap, and (3) vocational services must be rendered with the expectation that the individual will become gainfully employed. In most cases the majority of disabled students will meet all three eligibility requirements and, hence, involving BVR in the operations of a work-study program can be beneficial. An arrangement, then, must be made to refer students to BVR for determination of eligibility. The most efficient procedure is to have a BVR counselor assigned to a work-study program. The BVR counselor can

1. provide counseling on a one-to-one basis;
2. conduct home visits to obtain information on the student's family situation and coordinate the program with the family;
3. purchase needed student services such as work evaluation, work adjustment, medicals, psychiatric consultation, and psychological testing from the facility or other community resources;
4. provide placement and arrange on-the-job training for some students;
5. follow-up and continue to provide services to students who have been placed, and
6. provide needed feedback to the facility and school.

Liaison with School Personnel

To insure that both the work and the study aspects of the program are integrated, it is important to establish and maintain a strong working relationship with schoolteachers and administrators. Such a relationship is essential if (1) the facility's program is to benefit from the school's knowledge of the student and his problems, and (2) the school's instruction is to benefit from the facility's experience with the student. To avoid detachment of the two aspects of the program, channels of communication must be opened and school personnel must be encouraged to

1. provide basic background information on each student including academic performance, test scores, and special needs;
2. visit the home to coordinate the work-study program with

parents and work with the family in helping to resolve the student's problems;

3. visit the rehabilitation facility to observe how students are functioning at work, help identify and diagnose problem areas, and provide suggestions to the facility staff about how best to deal with group and individual problems, and

4. include, in school instruction, material suggested by the facility staff which will help students adapt to their new work experience. (This may include such things as the handling of money, the use of public transportation, standards of grooming and manners, and managing interpersonal relationships.)

Orientation of Students

Not only must the activities and services of the state agency and school be coordinated and integrated with those of the facility, but students must be oriented to the work part of the work-study program and motivated to seek its full benetfis. Hence, the student orientation to the facility is critical. The purpose of the initial orientation of students by the facility staff is to introduce facility and BVR staff that are involved, establish expectations and answer student questions. The actual orientation may consist of

1. the introduction of staff members, discussion of their relationships to the program and a description of their responsibilities;

2. discussion of goals of the work-study program;

3. discussion of the cooperative nature of the project between the school, rehabilitation facility, and state agency, and the services students can expect from each;

4. description of the various service programs (e.g. work evaluation) the student may experience, the rationale underlying the program and how it may be useful in the student's transition to work;

5. discussion of shop rules with emphasis on how these are similar to those encountered in industry;

6. assignment of students to facility rehabilitation staff coun-

selors and shop supervisors (a 10-15 ratio of students to re-habilitation staff is recommended);

7. a question and answer period for student inquiries.

Facility Services

This leads us to the actual service program the facility should be prepared to provide.* In addition to indirect or supportive services, these may include work evaluation, vocational and psychological testing, work adjustment, group counseling and training, work experience, and job seeking and placement services.

Work Evaluation

This is a dynamic, analytical process used to gather information concerning an individual's vocational potential. Evaluation is used to aid in vocational planning. A work evaluation program should provide an intensive work tryout experience in which counselors can observe how the student responds to instruction, how he learns to remember directions, how disabilities affect his work and the nature of his relationships with peers and supervisors. The environment in which this assessment is made is a rehabilitation workshop setting using simulated work tasks. The information gathered is integrated with other case history material by evaluators skilled in observation, diagnosis, and the understanding of personal and group dynamics.

There are basic questions that work evaluation is designed to answer:

1. Does the student possess the attitudes, interests, motivation and work goals necessary to launch into and benefit from a training program?

2. What is his current level of skill development, his manipulative, mechanical and clerical aptitudes, his work habits, such as punctuality and attendance, his mental and emotional stamina, his physical capacities?

3. How adequate is he in interpersonal relations, including relations with peers and supervisors?

---

* Parts of this section are adapted from O'Toole and Mather (1971), *Work Experience: Transition from School to Employment for Mentally Retarded Youth.*

4. Does he have the skills and other work requirements to enter into gainful or sheltered employment at the present time?
5. Can the individual learn, absorb instructions, and remember procedures?
6. Can he change sufficiently in the characteristics measured to become proficient after training?
7. Does he show strengths which will compensate for academic lacks or other deficiencies pictured in his medical, psychological, or vocational test findings?
8. What kind of rehabilitation program would be best suited to his needs and how can it be individually tailored to meet those needs?

The work evaluation process consists of about ten half-days of job sample testing. Briefly, work samples are systematically used to appraise work potential. A work sample is a close simulation of an actual industrial operation. The emphasis is not so much on present levels of ability but on ability to learn. Job sample categories may include bench assembly, academics (the utilization of time and money), clerical, sorting and categorizing, data processing, and sewing. A situational approach to work evaluation complements the work sample approach. It too is based upon the simulation of actual working conditions and work in the subcontract workshop. The student's current level of functioning, including his capacity for change, skill potential and social-emotional adjustment, is studied. Work evaluation is augmented by group counseling which is used for interpretive and diagnostic purposes and for observation of the student's behavior, ability to get along with peers, management of medications, attitudes toward supervision, and ability to take directions. Other rehabilitation professionals in the facility including physical therapists, occupational therapists, psychologists, psychiatrists, physicians, vocational counselors, educational specialists, work supervisors, and the shop's manager may also assist the work-evaluation counselor.

Vocational and Psychological Testing

Tests may be administered to the student by the facility's testing department, i.e. the Rotter Incomplete Sentence Blank, Purdue Pegboard, and the Minnesota Rate of Manipulation. In addition, each student may be given an intelligence test. Test results are analyzed in relation to the psychological tests furnished by the schools and the combined results are utilized in the interpretation of the student's work behavior and further refinements of his or her vocational plan.

Work Adjustment

A work adjustment phase of the work-study program may be initiated on the basis of work evaluation data and recommendations supplemented by information from the BVR counselor, the student's teachers, and data collected by the schools.* The two interrelated key elements in work adjustment are the rehabilitation workshop and the counselor who functions as a milieu therapist. The rehabilitation workshop is a simulated industrial work place where the student can learn and practice the various requirements of the work role. The counselor manipulates the workshop setting and uses individual and group counseling techniques to help the student become a productive worker. The goal of the work adjustment phase of the training is to develop within the student the attitudes and behavior patterns essential to employment. In addition, this may include efforts to improve work confidence and self-esteem; improve interpersonal relations between students and supervisors and students and their work peers; improve physical stamina, concentration, ability to remain with a work task, and improve grooming and dress.

The counselor's role is different from the traditional counseling role based on the medical-psychiatric model. Although the counselor does work with students in his office, when appropriate, he spends the great majority of his time out on the production floor working with groups and individuals. He is a participant in the work process and on the production floor where social distance which normally separates counselor and client is reduced.

The work situation is structured to maximize meaningful interaction between the student and the counselor. The counselor must be responsive to feedback from the student and use that

---

* See "A Situational Approach to Work Adjustment," Richard O'Toole and John L. Campbell (1971).

information in his further work with the student. The counselor is also in a position to observe the student's problems in the variety of situations which he confronts in the workshop setting. He can be there to assess behavior, suggest alternatives, and selectively reward behavior that is appropriate to the work role.

Much of the counselor's interaction with the student is concerned with defining the work role and showing the student how he can bring his behavior into the range acceptable by employers. The counselor utilizes situations that naturally arise in the work process, structures others to teach the value of work and encourages appropriate and discourages inappropriate behavior. He uses the routine of the workshop to teach punctuality, techniques to organize work, motion economy for increased production, the importance of following instructions and maintaining quality of work, acceptable behavior during coffee breaks, effective ways to communicate, and proper modes of movement in the work setting. Each of these will enable the student to maintain employment. Many of the counselor's efforts are especially directed toward leading the student to substitute adult-worker behavior for more immature and impulsive behavior. The counselor is there at the time clock, workbench, cafeteria, and in the halls with the student on a day-to-day basis to promote and support this change.

As a result of a long history of not doing well, many of the students are immobilized by low self-esteem and an accompanying fear of failure and need to develop a new view of themselves before they can begin to function well on the job. This can be accomplished in the work setting through the building of work confidence. By structuring the work setting so that the student can demonstrate ability, the counselor can build the base for a better self-image. The counselor must be sympathetic and understanding of failures and take every opportunity to help the student see his abilities. The counselor attempts to show the student ways to succeed in work and rewards the student in concrete ways for productive behavior. A sense of progress, efficacy, and accomplishment can be communicated to students in very concrete terms by using production charts which show progress toward competitive levels of productivity, increased wages, and promotion to more responsible positions in the work setting. These incentives encourage initiative and demonstrate that responsiveness to the demands of the work setting are rewarded. With greater confidence and a higher evaluation of himself as a result of progress on the job, the student's conception of work as another occasion for failure can be replaced with the knowledge that work can be a source of satisfaction and accomplishment.

The rehabilitation workshop presents many opportunities for evaluating and working with the student's problems in interpersonal relations on the job, especially problems with peers and supervisors. Using actual situations as they develop, the counselor may suggest ways of handling problems in a manner appropriate to the work setting, and point out the consequences of alternatives. Then, the student can learn and practice these new interpersonal skills under the guidance of the counselor.

The counselor can also enlist the aid of workshop supervisors and other students. Interpersonal relationships between students are an important source of motivation for change. Students, for example, can bring group pressure to bear to correct a peer's behavior. Similarly, their testimony of the fruitlessness of certain behaviors often has more validity than the counselor's injunction.

Another problem that students often bring to the facility involves the lack of physical stamina necessary to complete the work day. A student's physical capacity for work is a factor which must be carefully assessed. Strength, speed, and the ability to complete repetitious tasks for the full work day are especially important for the types of jobs in which disabled youth can be placed.

Similarly, a number of students have problems concentrating on a job or applying themselves productively for a sustained period of time. They may also not follow directions, indulge in diversions from work and not stick with a job until it is completed. One aim of the work adjustment process is to teach these individuals to stay with a task and maintain standards of quality and quantity of production. Again the counselor uses natural situations as they develop on the job as the basis for instruction.

The counselor can stimulate concentration by encouraging group efforts. By having work groups engage in controlled competition and by keeping group records of production, concentration and interest in the job can be enhanced.

Competition may be organized with rewards going to the most productive individuals or groups. Rewards may take the form of money, refreshments, and prestige of winning. In intergroup competition students can encourage one another and concentrate on using the most efficient procedures and techniques for the task at hand. The students will experience the meaning of teamwork and the part that the individual plays in work that requires the coordination of many individual's efforts. However, intra- and intergroup competition must be monitored and guided if its actions are not to be destructive. The work group, for example, can discriminate against those not able to contribute to group goals, and thus reinforce the student's poor evaluation of himself.

In addition to the problems directly related to work, many of the students have other problems. Working with the student and indirectly with his family, the counselor and other professionals must also attempt to deal with underlying medical and nutrition problems, living conditions, and life-styles which compromise the student's physical stamina. For example, many do not have an adequate conception of appropriate grooming and dress for the work role. A volunteer staffed grooming clinic may be beneficially developed to deal with these problems. Students can be taught appropriate dress, hair and skin care, and personal hygiene in general. Boys can be provided with grooming kits which include shoe polish, a razor, shaving cream, deodorant, a comb, and instructions on how to use them and why. Girls can be taken to a local vocational high school for a hair cutting, styling, shampooing and setting. More important, the counselor can define grooming standards and encourage and reward conformity to these standards.

Group Counseling

Group counseling sessions should be held frequently with the work shop director, vocational counselors, and BVR counselor assigned to a group. The purposes of group counseling are to help students to express their feelings, to learn how others deal with problems they may be experiencing, to find solutions to their own problems through open discussion, to gain insight into their behavior, and to acquire knowledge that enables them to move toward assumption of the work role. Subjects of discussion include problems concerning behavior at work, possible vocational goals, work attitudes, work quality, personal grooming, safety, honesty, and care of the work premises.

It may be of value to bring back a successfully employed former work-study student so that he can talk with the students in the group counseling sessions. He is not only an actual example of the success of the program in which they are involved but he can discuss his experiences on the job from a perspective much like their own.

Work Experience

In addition to subcontract work in the rehabilitation workshop, an effort should be made to design particular work experiences within the agency which are appropriate for this special group. Students can be assigned selectively and on a revolving basis to maintenance, reception, shipping and receiving, stock rooms, and tool rooms. They can also work as orderlies to assist physically handicapped clients, and on special occasions wait on customers and serve as coat checkers. This gives the student the chance to play the work role in new settings and helps him or her gain more work experience in different types of jobs. It also allows the staff to make evaluations in various jobs and settings. This broader range of work experience also helps the student in planning for the future because he can see to which type of work he seems to be the best suited. In one sense this phase of the work-study program is most like "on-the-job training."

Job Seeking Skills, Placement, and Follow-up

Depending on how the rehabilitation facility organizes the work-study program, placement services may be assigned to a school placement counselor, a rehabilitation placement counselor or to a BVR counselor. Basically, the student should receive some type of job-readiness training which involves discussion of employment opportunities, deduction of social security and withholding taxes, practice in filling out applications, and visits to prospective places of employment. Role-playing techniques and mock interviews with personnel directors in cooperating companies can be very helpful in preparing students for real interviews.

Students are normally placed during their senior year or during the summer following their graduation. However, many schools are now able to give credit to the student if he is employed prior to graduation, and this credit allows the student to graduate on time. Even after the student is placed, however, it must be recognized that the probabilities of continued successful employment are enhanced by follow-up and continued counselor support. The follow-up should last between three and twelve months, depending upon the student and the situation.

Administrative Problems

Thus far we have focused on the broad outlines of a work-study program for disabled youth. The program we have described has assumed that EMR's are the student population most likely to be encountered in the rehabilitation facility. In this section we look more closely at the kinds of organizational problems faced by the facility as it develops a work-study program.

Probably the single most important organizational problem facing the rehabilitation facility is the establishment of an ongoing sound source of program funding. Several possible sources of funds were identified earlier. Once this problem is solved, administrators can turn their attention to ongoing program management. The management problems attending the provision of rehabilitation services to disabled youth, especially those defined as EMR, derive from the age and disability characteristics of students, including the student's relationship with his family and the cooperative basis of the program, including the need to integrate the activities and expectations of state agency personnel, school personnel, students and parents, facility staff, and private industry.

Student Problems

In addition to problems associated with their disability, students in work-study programs will often bring with them a number of related and unrelated problems which effect their training and, if unresolved, affect their employability. In other words, a disabled youth is exposed to the influence of the family, school, and community as well as the agency. While participating in the program the students are confronted with problems which occur outside the agency but which must be dealt with by the agency if the client is to make any substantial progress toward his vocational goals. The counselor must be prepared to deal with these difficulties on a day-to-day basis, coordinate his activities with the student's teachers and parents, and enlist the services of other community agencies in an attempt to find solutions.

The child is taught work role behaviors in the family, school, and general community and sees them enacted by adults who act as role models. As he grows older, he is expected to take more responsibility for adequately organizing his various roles, such as his occupational role. Many disabled persons, however, are unable to do this. Having been defined as retarded, their families often do not expect them to be able to function in a responsible manner. Or, the student's family patterns may be incompatible with the work role. For example, the family may sleep late or require the young person to be around the home to run errands.

It is not the plan in the work-study program to change a student's style of life but to modify those particular habits which interfere with employment. Here we have in mind a broad spectrum of patterns which may need modification including everything from poor dietary habits to the timing and scheduling of activities throughout the day. Change must occur to allow the person to report to work on time and to engage in productive work for a full day. As with other problem areas, counselors deal with these difficulties on the spot, as they occur, and suggest concrete alternative courses of action.

There are several patterns of family life that may contribute to the student's disability and which tend to affect his work potential. One pattern that counselors have noted is the strict authoritarian father and the over-protective mother. Another is when, due to guilt or for other reasons, the family has not expected as much of the disabled child as they have of their other children. Some parents of disabled children seem unable to face the reality that the child must learn to make his own way. In these cases the child may lack confidence or be overly dependent on one or both parents. When, with advancing age, for example, parents come to realize that they have fostered dependency, patterns are often so deeply set they are intractable to rehabilitation methods.

Some students have grown up in homes where there were inappropriate or no worker role models from which behavior could be learned. Hence, as children they were not exposed to and did not learn work-related attitudes and behaviors. They often do not have aspirations which include employment, or those they do have may lack a sound basis in reality and experience. In other cases, the family's aspirations for the child may be completely beyond his capabilities.

Other conditions extraneous to the work-study program, but which influence the student's training and employability, include control of the student's idle time before and after work and during lunch and breaks, the student's inability to handle money and use public transportation, and parent reaction to wages and placement. Regarding the latter, many parents believe that their children should be earning more money for the work they do. Few parents are aware that it is legal to pay individuals less than the minimum wage. Hence, wage schedules must be interpreted and the possible benefits of Department of Labor guidelines must be explained. Similarly, efforts to place students outside the facility must be closely coordinated with parents, lest the parent not allow the student to continue on the job.

Organizational Problems

The most difficult problem facing the facility is the staffing of the program and the integration of its program with the school and its expectations, the industrial firms which provide contract work to the facility and employ the students after completion of the program, and the state agency and its requirements.

Problems that the rehabilitation facility face with its own staff may include recruiting counselors and other staff who are trained for work in such a program and the tendency for staff members to "burn out" after a few years of working closely with problem students. Because the staff is accountable for poor quality work produced by students and because the progress of many students is often slow, some staff members may lose their enthusiasm for this kind of work. Not surprisingly, there is a high turnover of staff in rehabilitation.

The problems which the facility may have with the schools include inability to obtain the student's permanent records; medical histories may be nonexistent or not current and recommendations may have been ignored; psychological tests may be outdated and/or lack any vocational interest inventories; certain disabilities may not be identified, and teachers may not be teaching material which is relevant to what is expected on a job, e.g. payroll checks, withholding taxes, bank accounts, piece rates, standard hours, and time clocks in hundredths of an hour. Further, teachers may not provide the needed feedback about the student and are difficult to reach in case of emergencies. Teachers often do not attend staffing conferences, and they usually have little knowledge of the community resources that the student can benefit from. Finally, once the student is placed in a rehabilitation facility, the school may be reluctant to take the student back, and problem students may have to be dealt with by the rehabilitation facility alone.

Industrial firm or economy related problems include keeping a steady flow of contract work into the rehabilitation facility, meeting delivery deadlines and quality standards, and coping with unforeseen problems such as strikes, fuel and material shortages, and economic slowdowns. Still other problems include competition from similar facilities, the tendency for some companies to encourage different rehabilitation facilities to bid against each other for the lowest price, and the resistance of some companies to hiring the handicapped. The former problems create financial burdens for the agency and the latter forces the agency to educate industrial firms in order to allay concern about insurance, architectural barriers, or the reactions of other employees to the new handicapped worker.

As with the school, problems with the state rehabilitation agency involve the difficulty of coordination. It is often difficult to keep the state agency counselor informed of student progress and because of the diffusion of responsibility and authority, there may be disagreements regarding the facility's recommendations. It may be noted that the school and family may also be involved. In any event, it becomes the responsibility of the facility to resolve differences when they occur.

These sets of problems suggest that a concordance of interests between the students and their parents and participating organizations and their staffs cannot be assumed. As the student, parent, school, rehabilitation agency, state agency and industrial firm are added to the equation, the number of interests and relationships that need to be accommodated proliferates. Further, the coordination of these interests and relationships is rendered expecially difficult by the fact that responsibility and authority are dispersed. An example will serve to illustrate the problems. Even if the recommendation of the facility staff is accepted by all principles and even if there are no organizational or program needs which compete with the student's needs (such as the need to fill a given training program), the facility, school and state agency may still disagree as to how the recommendations should be implemented. The facility may want to place the student into one of its training programs; the school may want to place the student into one of its manpower programs, and the state agency may want to place the student in an agency with which it has a contract. Because the student is leaving one of its programs, the burden is largely on the facility to ensure that the student's interests are held primary, and the various participants in the program do not work at cross purposes to these interests.

These problems of coordination, cooperation and accommodation are not insurmountable. It is important to point them out, however, because the success of a work-study program is fully dependent upon their resolution. When they are resolved, the work-study program can be an effective tool and students graduating from the program will be better equipped to enter the work force and contribute their independence and well-being not only to their firm but to society as well.

REFERENCES

Baller, W. R.: A study of the present social status of a group of adults, who, when they were in elementary schools, were classified as mentally deficient. *Genet Psychol Monogr, 18-19:*165-244, 1936-1937.

Beekman, M. E.: *The Retarded 200.* Lansing, Public Schools, 1963 (Mimeographed).

Bobroff, A.: Economic adjustment of 121 adults, formerly students in classes for the mental retardates. *Am J Ment Defic, 60:*525-535, 1956.

Charles, D. C.: Ability and accomplishment of persons earlier judged mentally deficient. *Genetic Psychol Monogr, 47:*3-71, 1953.

Jones, R., and Dyck, D.: Work-study programs: A survey of effectiveness. A comprehensive follow-up of work-study students in Montgomery County, Ohio, Montgomery County Board of Education. ESEA Title VI Project 51-MR-69. Ohio Department of Education, Division of Special Education, December, 1969.

Kolstoe, O. P., and Frey, R. M.: *A High School Work-Study Program for Mentally Subnormal Students.* Carbondale, Southern Illinois University Press, 1965.

McFall, T. M.: Postschool adjustment: A survey of fifty former students of classes for the educable mentally retarded. *Except Child, 32:*633-634, 1966.

O'Toole, R., and Campbell, J. L.: A situational approach to work adjustment. *J Rehabil, 37:*11-13, 1971.

O'Toole, R., and Mather, R. J.: *Work Experience: Transition from School to Employment for Mentally Retarded Youth.* Cleveland, Vocational Guidance and Rehabilitation Services, 1971.

Pavalko, R. M.: *Sociology of Education: A Book of Readings.* Ithaca, F. E. Peacock Publishers, 1968.

Phelps, H. R.: Postschool adjustment of mentally retarded in selected Ohio cities. *Except Child, XXIV*:410-412, 1958.

President's Committee on Employment of the Handicapped. *Employment of the Mentally Handicapped: A Group Discussion.* Washington, D. C., U. S. Government Printing Office, 1962.

Thomas, B. E.: A study of factors used to make a prognosis of social adjustments. *Am J Ment Defic, 47*:334-336, 1943.

Warren, F. G.: Kent county occupational and educational training project, progress report. Grand Rapids, Kent County Department of Special Education, Unpublished, 1963.

Wolfensberger, W.: Vocational preparation and occupation. In Baumeister, A. A. (Ed.): *Mental Retardation.* Chicago, Aldine Publishing, 1967.

Chapter 11

REHABILITATION FACILITIES FOR THOSE WITH SEIZURE DISORDERS

Leonard G. Perlman

The Problem

AMONG THE OLDEST AILMENTS known to man, epilepsy is still one of the world's least understood maladies. Epilepsy is a sign or symptom, not a disease, and results from or is part of an underlying neurological or systematic condition.

Epilepsy is often referred to as a convulsive disorder or cerebral dysrhythmia and always needs evaluation by a physician to determine the cause of the disturbance.

According to the Epilepsy Foundation of America (1972) an estimated 2 percent of the total U. S. population, or approximately four million people in the United States are believed to have some form of epilepsy.

While many persons with epilepsy are able to function adequately in society with the aid of anticonvulsant drugs, there are still a fair proportion whose needs for proper diagnosis, treatment and rehabilitative services are not being met.

Wright (1965) indicates that "even when seizures are controlled, psychological and environmental problems frequently create several personal difficulties for the epileptic. Family feelings of guilt and fear which often lead to indulgence and overprotection, may limit healthy emotional growth and adjustment. Combine this with the problems of rejection by others in school, the neighborhood, and places of employment, and the dilemma of a multi-handicapped individual emerges.

Unfortunately, far too many persons with seizure disorders are not benefitting from recent medical advances and those in the social and vocational areas. This serious factor illuminates the pressing need for comprehensive facilities which will specialize in providing services to persons with epilepsy.

Wright goes on to say that successful rehabilitation requires the expert knowledge of members of a multidisciplinary team to work with all aspects of the individual. This is especially important in epilepsy because of the complex interaction of life adjustment and medical control problems.

Facilities, if they are to be effective, must link together the skills of community medicine and social and rehabilitation approaches. While this statement is certainly not novel, this approach in the rehabilitation of those with convulsive disorders has not been exploited nearly enough. Yet the evidence for a comprehensive, multidisciplinary effort can be clearly delineated.

Trends in Facilities for Those with Epilepsy

The general trend in the United States has been to close the twelve or thirteen epilepsy colonies which existed as the main inpatient resource solely for those with epilepsy. Only the New Castle State Hospital in Indiana currently remains operational. In addition, only one facility exists for youth of average intellectual potential with seizure disorders who are also experiencing social and emotional difficulties. This is the National Children's Rehabilitation Center located in Leesburg, Virgina. This setting provides a multidisciplinary approach which stresses medical management of seizures, special education, counseling, psychotherapy and emphasis on group living procedures.

In general, the only type of inpatient facilities available to those with epilepsy are state hospitals and training schools for the mentally retarded and state hospitals for the mentally ill. In these settings, however, the primary disability is usually mental retardation and emotional disturbance, respectively. Specialized facilities for those with epilepsy as a primary problem do not exist in the U. S. except for the two settings previously mentioned (Indiana and Virginia).

The Neurological and Sensory Disease Control Program (NSDCP) of the Public Health Service which operated between 1962 and 1970 named epilepsy as a primary area of concern. Cereghino and Cole (1970) indicated that the NSDCP was concerned with the multidisciplinary approach to improve services for persons with epilepsy. This was undertaken through studies, service demonstration grants, training grants and educational and informational activities. Cereghino and Cole revealed that a total of twenty-five multidisciplinary demonstration clinics were funded from 1963 to 1970. One of their significant findings was that the "Rehabilitation of hard-core epileptics not reached by previous treatment methods is possible through the multidisciplinary approach." A demonstration program of note was carried out at the Barrow Neurological Institute and clearly proved the feasibility and the need for this type of approach in the rehabilitation and habilitation of persons with epilepsy. Fundamental objectives included multidisciplinary case finding, diagnosis, treatment, and follow-up services where these were not currently available. According to Cereghino and Cole, the method used was to "encourage the development of specialized regional programs for convulsive disorders in broad-based community, regional, or statewide demonstration projects.

Cole (1965) listed the criteria developed by NSDCP in stimulating and evaluating community demonstration projects as follows:

1. Availability of medical and teaching centers as a resource for skilled medical manpower and technology.
2. Potential for further development of regional or satellite clinics for referral and follow-up; usually a community hospital.
3. Effective liaison with state and local health departments and voluntary health agencies.
4. Recognition of the importance of continuing education for physicians in the diagnosis and management of epilepsy.
5. A community-based organization to provide information on epilepsy for lay and professional groups.
6. Potential for future expansion of epilepsy service to a broader diagnostic and evaluation neurological service.

By 1970, or the time of the completion of the NSDCP demonstration projects, two types of clinics emerged: (1) *A regional center* which included complete evaluative services, where research and services were closely interwoven and where professional and public education could be undertaken, and (2) *A network of satellite clinics* throughout an area served and staffed by personnel from a central clinic.

Ideally, a combination of the above would provide the best possible coverage for the patient and include staffs from professions such as a neurology, psychology, rehabilitation counseling, social work, nursing, electroencephalograph (EEG) technology, and education.

Another project of note was conducted at the Kenny Institute of Minneapolis under a grant by the Vocational Rehabilitation Administration (HEW). This study demonstrated the improvement in the employment potential of persons with epilepsy when comprehensive rehabilitation methods are coordinated. de Torres (1962) reported on the procedures used at the Institute which included detailed patient and family interviews, neurological examinations, EEG studies, psychological tests, school and employment histories and a review of health and welfare agency files. Next, case staffing was held to recommend and plan for the rehabilitative course of action for each patient. Techniques applied included pre-vocational workshop evaluations (when needed), patient and family counseling, group therapy, work adjustment training, and job placement. The significant findings by de Torres included that 61.5 percent of 102 patients were capable of competitive employment and that this factor could be traced to the effectiveness of the multidisciplinary team.

From the data presented thus far it is most encouraging that those with convulsive disorders, once wrote off as hopeless, can benefit from a well-coordinated team of professional disciplines operating out of a comprehensive setting.

European Facilities

Several European countries have specific treatment facilities for those with epilepsy needing inpatient care and an array of rehabilitative services.

The Netherlands, for example, has three special centers for

epilepsy with a bed capacity of 1,250 and eight outpatient clinics. According to Meinardi (1972) there is currently a shift in these centers from nursing home care to a total rehabilitation program with an emphasis on the multidisciplinary team approach. The orientation is the development of the individual to his highest medical, social and employment potential. The need for special facilities for those with epilepsy is described by Meinardi who stated that while there are several clinical entities of epilepsy, many with epilepsy have similar features in common and that the uncertain relationship between the type of epilepsy and the medication to be prescribed demands lengthy trials. This is expecially true in viewing the gradual build-up of effective blood levels for the control of seizures. Meinardi stated that if the epileptic patient cannot obtain freedom from attacks on an outpatient basis, that a special center that offers schooling as well as vocational training be available. He cites an additional advantage in the facilities concept in that bringing together persons with epilepsy provides a therapeutic milieu where patients under comparable circumstances can be carefully observed for reactions to anticonvulsants. This has obvious value from a research point of view.

The goals of special centers were listed by Meinardi as follows:

1. Suppression of seizures with the least possible side effects.
2. Restoration of optimal social relationships.
3. Vocational rehabilitation.

While the Netherlands approach utilizes special centers for epilepsy treatment and rehabilitation, they also stress the strong link of the outpatient department in returning the patient to productive life in the community. The epilepsy center here is viewed as a temporary setting to prepare patients for independent living and that permanent care be delegated to nursing homes or halfway houses.

Henriksen (1972) reports that Norway has a National Hospital for epileptics at Sandvika, which consists of a multidisciplinary staff of physicians, psychologists, social workers, teachers and nurses. This 180-bed facility has a rehabilitation section, laboratories for biochemical and neurophysiological examinations and research, and two homes for chronic epileptics. The services provided by this facility is similar to those found in Norway and are listed as follows:

1. Diagnosis
2. Adjustment of medication requiring a biochemical laboratory
3. Selection for surgical treatment, requiring a neurophysical laboratory
4. Psychological and psychiatric treatment
5. Schooling and rehabilitation
6. Aftercare services
7. Outpatient services
8. Research capability
9. Information services
10. Education of medical personnel

Henriksen indicated that in Norway the total number of patients in need of life-long observation is estimated at 200 per year, as a minimal figure. This coupled with the importance of patients remaining as close to their communities as possible has given rise to the proposed plan to have special epilepsy centers connected to four university hospitals in Norway.

England currently has ten institutions which provide residential care for approximately two thousand persons with epilepsy. Seven of these settings are considered "colonies" and were built between 1888 and 1905. Reid (1972) reports that while the original concept of such a colony was largely a self-supporting rural community with little emphasis on vocational training, the trend in recent years is toward active rehabilitation. Reid relates that while the old colony concept fulfilled a valuable role in the past, as newer techniques in diagnosis and treatment continue to improve, there should be a steady reduction in those requiring long-term care. The trend in England, as in other nations, has been toward community care, however, it is also recognized that for some, residential care on a long-term basis is a necessity.

Lund (1972) described the Filadelphia Colony as the only major center for epileptics in Denmark. This colony with four associated nursing homes had 130 patients who had been hospitalized from zero to twelve months. Lund reported that 55 percent of the beds in the Filadelphia Colony are occupied by patients who have been there for at least one year.

In conclusion, Lund recommends that an epilepsy center should accept patients of all ages and with all types and degrees of epilepsy as well as the most severe cases. In order to avoid "mental and social institutionalization," however, Lund sees the need for day care centers for those disabled living at home, residential care for severe cases, protected hostels (equivalent to group foster home care), and "specially protected workshops" (sheltered workshops) for those with poor work skills or those unable to compete in the labor market.

In 1972 a multidisciplinary center opened near Brussels in Belgium. Known as the William Lennox Center for Epilepsy, it was planned to take into account a wide array of patient needs from treatment via the family physician through a multidisciplinary, outpatient clinic or residential care clinic. The center emphasized the most modern neurophysiological and rehabilitative approaches. To this end, workshops and training centers, schools and playing fields are seen as important aspects of the facility. The Lennox Center is the result of twenty years of planning based on findings of more than fifty institutions throughout the world.

Projected Programs in the United States

In the U. S., although widely discussed and studied for many years, the comprehensive epilepsy center is just recently coming closer to operational reality. The National Institute for Neurological Diseases and Stroke (NINDS) of the Department of Health, Education and Welfare developed guidelines in 1973 for the development of centers. Its objective, according to the *National Spokesman* (July-August 1973) is to provide "complete services for all patients with epilepsy within a defined geographic area and population, and to be achieved by effectively coordinating and, when indicated, extending existing services."

This approach was outlined in the *National Spokesman* as follows:

Direct Services

The program will ensure that complete up-to-date preventive, medical, rehabilitative, psychological, and social services are provided to people with epilepsy, such as:

—*Early recognition and diagnosis,* involving case findings, perhaps through screening and total assessment of needs.

—*Social, educational and vocational rehabilitation,* including protective and legal services, sheltered employment and recreation.

—*Information and referral services* to patients and physicians, including follow-up services.

—*Long-term residential care* at all levels, such as custodial, half-way houses, foster homes, or group homes.

—*Transportation services* necessary to assure access to services.

—A *detailed registry* of all patients in a geographic area.

The NINDS guidelines indicate that although centers would bear the responsibility for developing the total program, not all services would originate in one place. For example, sheltered workshops and residential centers are cited as service facilities that could be located elsewhere. If this turns out to be the case, then the centers set up by the program would differ somewhat from their European counterparts, where all services are usually concentrated in one location.

Physical Plant

The guidelines also deal with the physical components of a future center and it would consist of the following:

—Outpatient facilities and satellite clinics;

—Complete inpatient diagnostic and hospitalization facilities;

—Research facilities and laboratories;

—Facilities for education, vocational training and employment;

—Long-term residential care, psychological and family counseling, and other social services.

These centers are patterned after other rehabilitation and treatment centers for cancer, heart and stroke, and also those designed to deal with a variety of disability categories.

This total approach to rehabilitation and habilitation, which has been in the planning and demonstration stages for many years, should bring the person with convulsive disorders closer to leading a more productive life.

Summary

The trend in the U. S. is toward comprehensive community health care delivery systems. The focus is to keep the patient in or close to his community, or, if institutionalized, to return the individual to the home environment as soon as possible. These admirable goals have not been implemented on a wide scale for certain handicapping conditions. Unfortunately, for those with a primary disability of epilepsy, comprehensive services at the community level have not been easy to locate. In addition, inpatient facilities for care and rehabilitation specifically for those with seizure disorders are virtually nonexistent in the U. S. today. For these reasons, persons with epilepsy are not receiving the full benefits from recent medical advances and improved rehabilitation procedures.

The multidisciplinary approach has proven to be the most effective method as evidenced by projects in both the U. S. and Europe. While prevention and cure or total control of all seizures may not be in sight, significant medical and rehabilitative approaches are available. These advances must be brought together in a system of comprehensive rehabilitation centers that provide a broad array of services designed to maximize the potential of those with convulsive disorders.

The newest of the European multidisciplinary centers opened in 1972 in Brussels, Belgium. It is known as the William Lennox Center for Epilepsy. This facility emphasizes the latest in modern neurophysiological and rehabilitative approaches and includes outpatient and residential care, vocational workshops, training centers and recreation programs.

The current trend in the United States is to build upon the demonstrated effectiveness of the multidisciplinary approaches explored by the federal government, private and voluntary agencies over the past three decades. Most recently, the National Institute of Neurological Diseases and Stroke (NINDS), one of the National Institutes of Health, has developed guidelines for feasibility studies for comprehensive epilepsy centers. The coordinated services needed for such facilities include medical, psychological and social services and involve the following specific aspects:

1. early recognition and diagnosis,
2. social, educational and vocational rehabilitation including vocational workshops,
3. information and referral services including follow-up care,
4. long-term residential care including custodial, halfway houses, foster care or group homes,
5. transportation to assure access to services, and
6. a detailed registry of all patients in a given geographic location.

While the center would be responsible for developing the total program, not all services would eminate from one location; sheltered workshops or halfway houses could be located elsewhere within the geographical boundaries of the center.

The many agencies and organizations involved with this concept would include the following: medical institutions, educational facilities, research facilities and laboratories, employment facilities such as sheltered and transitional workshops, local public agencies such as the vocational rehabilitation office, and the private voluntary agency. The latter being the Epilepsy Foundation of America which currently serves as the spokesman and advocate for those with seizure disorders in the United States.

While the growth of rehabilitation facilities in the United States has been phenomenal the comprehensive service needs for those with epilepsy has not as yet seen any sustained national effort. This latest movement to develop comprehensive services is anticipated with much hope for those who have gone far too long without adequate attention—the person with epilepsy.

REFERENCES

Cereghino, J. J., and Cole, C. H.: A multidiciplinary approach to services for the epileptic. *Health Services and Mental Health Services Report,* 86:4, 1971.
Cole, C. H.: The Role of the U. S. Public Health Services Bureau of State

Services in Epilepsy Control. From a Symposium on Epilepsy, Madison, University of Wisconsin, November 5, 1965.

de Torres, T. *et al.: Employment Problems of Epileptics.* Minneapolis, E. Kennedy Institute, 1962.

Directory of rehabilitation facilities. *J Rehabil, 34:*4, 1968.

Henriksen, G. F.: Special centers in the Netherlands. *Epilepsia, 4:*13, 1972.

Lund, M.: Special centers in the Netherlands. *Epilepsia, 4:*13, 1972.

Meinardi, H.: Special centers in the Netherlands. *Epilepsia, 4:*13, 1972.

National Spokesman. Belgium, Epilepsy Centers 6, 9, 1973.

Recognition, Onset, Diagnosis Therapy. Epilepsy Foundation of America, 1972.

Reid, J. J. A.: Special centers in the Netherlands. *Epilepsia, 4:*13, 1972.

Wright, G. N.: Progress report on epilepsy. *J Rehabil, 21:*6, 1965.

CHAPTER 12

THE NEEDS OF SPINAL CORD INJURED CLIENTS IN SHELTERED WORKSHOPS

ROBERT A. LASSITER

SHELTERED WORKSHOP administrators are aware of the progress that has been made in medical science, technology and practice during the past three decades which has contributed to the development of a broad and comprehensive approach in rehabilitation for people with spinal cord injuries. Since World War II, physical medicine and rehabilitation as practiced in public and private facilities has demonstrated that the impact of paraplegia and quadraplegia need not be catastrophic. When the medical and paramedical services for this group proved to be successful, vocational evaluation became an important element in the total rehabilitation process. But, as long as spinal cord injuries were considered catastrophic and resulted in profound disablement or death, vocational implications were not explored in workshops. Thus, it can be seen that sheltered workshop services for this disability group represent relatively new concerns (Savine, Belchick and Brean, 1971).

Physical medicine and rehabilitation departments in hospitals, rehabilitation centers and workshops now accept general responsibility for dealing with the vocational implications of spinal cord injury. Physiatrists usually agree that rehabilitation "involves treatment and training of the patient to the end that he may attain his maximum potential for normal living physically, psychologically, socially and vocationally" (Krusen, Kottke, and Ellwood, 1966). This way of viewing the total person and his needs is unique in medicine. The emphasis on the vocational implications creates a climate of acceptance for the work evaluator and work adjustment person in the workshop setting which is not found when these people work with physicians in other areas of disability. However, this same acceptance places great demands on the vocational rehabilitation staff: the vocational problems added to an already complicated and complex disability may produce serious anxiety and frustration on the part of the workshop staff because of the lack of an organized and systematic approach in viewing the vocational implications of this disability.

The purpose of this chapter is to explore the vocational needs or deficits that are experienced by people who suffer a spinal cord injury and, in this way, to identify for administrations and staff of workshop programs the nature of the implications that are peculiar to people with this disability. A review of the more recent trends and development in workshop programs and a series of interviews with people with spinal cord injuries indicates that the major needs expressed by patients or clients appear to be equal in significance to those observed by all rehabilitation practitioners. It appears these needs can best be identified by relating them to Maslow's formulation of his motivation theory: the arrangement of basic needs in a hierarchy of less or greater priority or potency: physiological, safety, belongingness and love, esteem and self-actualization (Maslow, 1970).

Perhaps this approach to a study of vocational needs of severely handicapped people will, at times, be indistinguishable from psychological or social studies or frames of reference. This appears unavoidable, however, if we are to accept any categorization since needs that are called vocational are never independent of the physical, psychological or social needs of people with severe physical limitations, but are intertwined with all other basic needs. In his exploration of broad categories of needs related to work, Walter Neff has provided a category of needs specific to work which correspond with Maslow's basic need list: material needs, self-esteem, activity, respect by others, and the need for creativity. In the following consideration of the vocational implications of cord injuries, Neff's statements reflect the views expressed in the listing of the five hierarchical needs that "the problems of work behavior are, in large part at least, problems of personality" (Neff, 1968).

Physiological Needs

Remarkable advances in medical treatment and care of paraplegics and quadraplegics have contributed to a greater awareness of the physical needs related to work adjustment. The basic physiological needs of the person with a spinal cord injury are apparent: to survive from a major trauma to the body involves the person in a schedule of nutrition, using drugs to fight infection, undergoing surgical procedures and strict adherence to a program in muscle redevelopment and reeducation. Much emphasis in the rehabilitation medicine program is in the teaching of the patient the basic survival physical skills which he or she acquired earlier as an infant or child. In addition to this reeducation or redevelopment phase, there is also a need for a new skill to be taught to accommodate the new physical limitations —to learn new methods in self-care and mobility. These lead to the "activities of daily living" therapeutic aspects of the physical medicine program.

But, what are the vocational limitations which help the person meet his physiological needs beyond medical and paramedical therapy? There are major physical needs with significance for sheltered workshop staff in a work adjustment program.

Need to Learn to Work in a Wheelchair

To work in a wheelchair is the most obvious physical need rather than to be limited in occupational choice because of inability to walk or run on the job if paraplegia is the case, or limited by the inability to use hands and arms in the usual way in the case of quadraplegia. In addition, movement from home to the shop and from one position in the work setting to another, e.g. using the rest room, taking a coffee break, meeting with fellow workers or trainees, are all movements on the job that non-disabled people make without conscious effort while attending to the demands of a job. In mobility problems such as these, clients in vocational evaluation and work adjustment programs must consider also the travel barriers including automobile parking problems as well as a variety of architectural barriers from steps to the too narrow doors for wheelchairs which are still observed in some workshops.

Need to Learn New Ways of Being Productive

Many times it is necessary that vocational planning include a work time schedule different from other clients but maintaining the same production goals. Special structural pieces and instruments enable the client to meet the job demands, e.g. a "raised platform or a lowered machine"; and, at times, the designation of one worker as a person who can stand by to assist the client in meeting certain physical needs of an emergency nature including critical problems with bladder and bowel and safety concerns such as the use of a ramp caked with ice and snow. It is important that these kinds of needs be met with a goal of assisting the client toward independence, rather than building dependency type relationships. Some clients can accept a lot of help and a dependent role; others, however, can accept help only if absolutely required for survival. There is a great need for the client to receive an individualized instructional program in mobility in the workshop and acceptance of help from others in order to cope with the physical limitations imposed by spinal cord injury.

Need for the Client to Accept Responsibility for Personal Hygiene

The client must learn skills in medical and therapeutic areas beyond the basic physical needs of following good health habits which apply to the non-disabled person. For good health all people are concerned with good nutrition, adequate sleep and rest, and regular physical checkups. However, able-bodied workers can "get away" with some abuses to the body, at least temporarily, while the person with cord injury cannot "let go"; he has a continuing need to follow the regular habits of good health, plus!

The person who has a spinal cord injury and works as a client in a workshop setting is able to be productive only when he learns to live his life well and move about in a wheelchair, attend to toilet and other personal needs, to adapt to new ways toward independence by acceptance of special assistance such as modification of the work environment and "emergency" dependence on one other person on the job. And above all, he must give his maximum effort to care for his body and avoid the medical complications and intercurrent illnesses, which result in absenteeism, loss of productive activity and more severe disablement.

Safety Needs

Following Maslow's conceptual framework, the person with a cord injury, once having met the physical needs, perceives new needs emerging in terms of personal safety. Here the client is concerned with his security and stability, freedom from fear, anxiety and chaos, and his personal protection. Some of the needs that become dominant at this point in vocational planning overlap with physical needs. Because of the severity of the disability, the physical needs may not ever be well gratified. Major vocational implications observed in this need are the strong desire on the part of the individual to remain in work that is similar to his previous job and a preference for association with people on the job who are familiar to him and the need for a job which appears to offer greater tenure and stability with better than average health and retirement plans. There is a need felt for a smoothly functioning position with order clearly established. The healthy appeal of innovation change and adventure may no longer surface. As Maslow states, "The threat of chaos or of nihilism can be expected in most human beings to produce a regression from any higher needs to the more prepotent safety needs" (Maslow, 1970). Thus, there is a strong possibility that the individual experiencing the constant threat to physical health may look to an authoritative or military type organization for this "protection" he seeks.

Workshop program planning, then, must consider the possible "security and stability" needs that may be directly attributable to the spinal cord injury or may be the consequences of changes to the person and his life circumstances. Otherwise, following the severe trauma of the injury, the individual may stabilize finally in the role of invalid with some welfare or other compensation program, become semiretired, or a permanent resident of the workshop (Kutner, 1968).

Belongingness and Love Needs

When the members of the rehabilitation workshop team are able to help the client meet the physical and safety needs in a satisfactory way, the emphasis in coping involves love and affection or belongingness needs. For the first time in his life, the person with a cord injury may "feel sharply the pangs of loneliness, of ostracism, of rejection, of friendlessness, of restlessness" (Maslow, 1970). This need to love and be loved has been stressed by all theorists of psychology and there is much clinical evidence showing that the thwarting of love needs is basic in the picture of maladjustment, as shown by Maslow. However, love and affection as well as their possible expression in sexuality, are generally looked upon with some reluctance by the workshop staff. And in many instances, sexual needs, if considered at all, are associated with despair and hopelessness.

In addition to these more obvious problems, love and affection needs may not realistically be met by the staff nor by a job. Thus, a problem arises for the client and the workshop staff: how is instruction and counseling that can help the client find new ways of developing feelings of belongingness, to be loved and to love, or, in some cases, to maintain the ability to love and be loved provided? Much more emphasis is being given in centers today, and a few articles are seen such as "Sex and Spinal Cord Injured Male" by a physician in a recent issue of *Paraplegia News.* Also, some success in meeting this need may be found by the client as he participates in one of the rapidly developing encounter or sensitivity training sessions whose members work in small groups to fight alienation and loneliness and seek belongingness or togetherness in the "face of a common enemy."

Perhaps, through participation in personal growth groups with people without cord injuries, clients can find opportunities for practicing "loving and being loved." Despite the difficulty faced by rehabilitation staff members in helping the client meet this important need, success on the future job will depend, to some extent, on this need being met. Workshop personnel can assist by carefully analyzing the potential for caring and being cared for which may be provided in a particular job setting.

The Esteem Needs

People with cord injuries have a great need for self-esteem as well as esteem from others, just as all people do. Maslow refers to Alfred Adler's work in his summary of the basic elements of the esteem needs: "the desire for strength, for achievement, for adequacy, for mastery and competence, for confidence in the face of the world, and for independence and freedom (self-esteem) and, second, we have the desire for reputation, or prestige, status, dominance, recognition, attention, importance, etc. (respect or esteem from other people) (Maslow, 1970).

There is an opportunity in sheltered workshops to provide training programs for the client to develop skills needed to meet the esteem needs. The client is able to experience new feelings of competence and self-confidence that come from a person's exposure to new interpersonal skills and new tasks which are individually selected based on the client's inner nature and perception of self. Karen Horney states "out of one's Real Self rather than out of the idealized pseudo-self" and, to avoid the dangers of "having self-esteem on the opinions of others rather than on real capacity, competence and adequacy to the task" (Maslow, 1970).

Workshop adjustment plans for people with cord injuries must include a variety of approaches which can meet these esteem needs. An ideal program will give priority to meeting these needs through activities such as specific work task assignments, individual counseling, and using small group encounter sessions with a combination of affective and cognitive activities. The workshop staff will need to differentiate the good self-esteem feelings received from actual competence as experienced by the client from the external, sometimes artificial and forced supportive counseling which leaves the client with low esteem feelings from both self and others. Also, it is important to individualize the approach because of the uniqueness of each individual who has suffered cord injury. Some people at the onset of disability have already received the "blessings" of esteem and may cope in this area better than those whose injury occurred before these esteem needs were met.

The work adjustment staff person in the workshop has the responsibility for analyzing the individual client's characteristics in order to have a basis for selecting the methods that are most relevant to meeting his or her needs. Some clients may need opportunities to explore ways of developing or re-developing self-esteem needs through the type of work and interpersonal encounters that are provided in "milieu therapy." As defined by Kutner, the environment of a workshop setting is utilized as a training ground for patients to exercise social and interpersonal skills and to test their ability to deal with both simple and complex problems commonly experienced in open society. The treatment program attempts to engage the patient in various social encounters; these experiences provide tests of judgment, of social competences, of problem-solving ability, and of social responsibility. Milieu therapy must attempt to provide the patient with an arsenal of skills to overcome frustration with enlightened self-interest and high morale (Kutner, 1968).

This particular approach offers the client a wide range of activities to experience personal growth for meeting esteem needs which are in some ways different from the approaches used to assist the client in the belongingness needs. For example, the use of social encounters in meeting the esteem needs are related to the exploration of vocational interests and abilities and the demonstration of work behaviors and work attitudes which can be observed by the staff.

An extensive study made at the University of North Carolina in Chapel Hill indicates the need for rehabilitation personnel to present to the client a framework for ordering a period of socialization. Cogswell reports that the five year study of paraplegics from injury and hospitalization to return to the community showed that most paraplegics who eventually resume work roles delay for one to several years and, that returning paraplegics had a marked reduction in the number of social contacts with others, frequency in entering community settings and the number of roles they played. To counteract this problem, she recommends that rehabilitation staffs can help to close this gap by guiding clients through the steps of socialization in workshop settings. The study also indicated that initial stalling by the paraplegics is in no way predictive of job success or failure. This recommendation for an active assistance plan for socialization runs parallel with other reports that show the need for people with cord injuries to continue to have some contact over a longer time with rehabilitation facility staff (Cogswell, 1968).

The Need for Self-Actualization

Maslow uses the term self-actualization as it refers to man's desire for self fulfillment, namely, "to the tendency for him to become actualized in what he is potentially . . . the desire to become more and more what one idiosyncratically is, to become everything that one is capable of becoming . . . and, the clear emergence of these needs (self-actualization) rests upon some prior satisfaction of the physiological, safety, love and esteem needs" (Maslow, 1970).

Just as in other needs that the cord injured person must meet, this one may be met partially, at least, through a sound work adjustment program in the sheltered workshop. It is important, though, that consideration be given to the uniqueness of the individual. Some people seem to have greater self-actualization needs than others. Many people may not experience a desire for self-actualization nor feel frustrated in not receiving gratification of this need; while all other needs appear to be important or necessary for good work adjustment, there may be no feeling of frustration about this need. "In certain people the level of aspiration may be permanently deadened or lowered . . . the less prepotent goals may simply be lost, and may disappear forever, so that the person who has experienced life at a very low level (chronic unemployment or severe limitations from disability), may continue to be satisfied for the rest of his life if only he can get enough food" (Maslow, 1970).

It appears here that the implication for vocational planning is dependent, then, on the individual's special need for self-actualization. If the cord injured person has been successful in coping with life, and the other four needs were met in a fairly satisfactory way in the rehabilitation process, it is possible the client will indicate a strong desire to seek a work environment in which he can find opportunities for spontaniety, purpose in work behavior (mission in life), autonomy on the job, and innovation and creativeness. Certain workshop professional staff who read this part of the text may be able to identify with these desires for a job that allows for genuine self-actualization, as defined by Maslow. However, these same readers can also appreciate that they may be in the minority. As Neff states, "Only a small number of people in modern society are fortunate enough to find in their work an opportunity to create something genuinely expressive of their unique qualities" (Neff, 1968). For many people participating in a workshop program, there may be a need for the development of innate creative skills that will become leisure time activities and any perceived self-actualization needs will be met through avocations or hobbies, rather than through a job.)

In preparation for this writing, the author visited Woodrow Wilson Rehabilitation Center in Fishersville, Virginia and interviewed six people who are seriously affected by spinal cord injury. The questions posed to each client were related to what the client considered to be the strongest vocational implications of the disability. Either physical and safety needs, or love and belongingness needs, or esteem needs were discussed by one or more of the clients but, only one of the needs, self-actualization, was articulated by all six people. Obviously, this was not the language or jargon chosen by the clients to express this particular need; however, in each interview the client spoke to this need in responses such as "I need a new faith in myself, now"; "I want good feelings in my abilities as a person"; "I am discovering within myself a new richness of life"; "I want to keep learning from him (a television evangelist) about what my life means"; "I want to give to life, rather than just take." These responses were accompanied in most instances with a discussion about opportunities for positive changes in life's direction as a result of the disability. Victor Frankl might refer to these statements as representative of the existential anxiety experienced by people in trouble and the need for a spiritual element in therapy for people who have suffered some catastrophic event.

In rehabilitation, this basic need of many clients, self-actualization, has been left to each individual to work out, for the most part. It appears that consideration should be given to what John Wax calls "a new dimension of rehabilitation" in workshop programs. Wax reviews the two primary themes of rehabilitation. These are, traditionally, achievement and interaction which he states are necessary, but may not be sufficient. He then goes on to discuss the idea of the possibility of a third dimension being added to the rehabilitation process:

> There is a possibility of a third dimension or a third major value for the disabled, namely, the development of the inner life, inner resources, or inner space. . . . Of course the vast majority of clients are very action-oriented, and few are inclined to be introspective. This is not to suggest that we train active patients to sit around and contemplate their navels, but there are some people who should be offered the option no matter how busy most of us continue to be, there comes a time when we must be alone and face our existential loneness . . . for many, being alone is synonymous with boredom, alienation, loneliness, isolation, abandonment or exile (Wax, 1972).

Wax presents four major reasons for assisting seriously handicapped people in a self-awareness and self-actualization program: (1) a rich inner life may make being alone less painful; (2) inner space (or thought) may be the only area left for a feeling of freedom and autonomy for those who are dependent on others; (3) effective use of this inner space (being happy with your thoughts and feelings) offers an alternative to the hyperactivity of people who fear depression or existential despair, and (4) solitude and the ability to think and ask ourselves the hard questions give us the opportunity to develop a philosophy which helps us to live what must be lived, e.g. a life of severe disability. "A philosophy which helps us to find meaning and purpose can be enormously useful" (Wax, 1972).

Techniques recommended for workshop personnel which meet this self-actualization need of people with cord injuries might include activities such as meditation, Gestalt awareness, alpha feedback, use of fantasies and daydreams, and other self-awareness exercises that can be provided either in individual or group counseling. An awareness of this need for self-actualization on the part of the client is the first step for the rehabilitation worker to take; the second step is to determine the unique way this need is to be met by the person, and the third is to provide the opportunity for activities in the workshop that will enhance the vocational adjustment of the client. As the authors of "Disability, Rehabilitation and Existentialism" state, "Existentialism encourages the patient to grow beyond mere adjustment, to reject societal interpretations of his disability, and to continue the creative life . . . if there is meaning to suffering, there is also an opportunity for the patient to transcend that suffering and live every moment of his existence to the fullest extent" (Easton and Krippner, 1964).

Summary

Following a brief statement on the background of this severe disability, the vocational implications for people with cord injuries were discussed. Maslow's hierarchy of need theory was used as a basis for exploring the special needs of people with cord injuries in sheltered workshop settings. In each of the needs in the hierarchy, physiological, safety, belongingness, esteem and self-actualization, an effort was made to demonstrate these basic needs as the five major vocational implications and to offer suggestions for sheltered workshop staff on ways of assisting clients in moving toward freedom and independence in work adjustment and eventually in outside satisfactory employment, when possible.

REFERENCES

Cogswell, Betty E.: Self socialization: Readjustment of paraplegics in the community. *J Rehabil, 34*:3, 1968.

Dreikurs, Rudolph: *Fundamentals of Adlerian Psychology.* Chicago, Alfred Adler Institute, 1953.

264   *Rehabilitation Facility Approaches*

Easton, Harry, and Krippner, Stanley: Disability, rehabilitation, and existentialism. *Personnel and Guidance Journal, 43:3,* 1964.

Hohmann, George W.: Sex and the spinal cord injured male. *Paraplegia News,* February, 1973.

Horney, Karen: *Neurosis and Human Growth.* New York, Norton, 1950.

Kutner, Bernard: Milieu therapy in rehabilitation medicine. *J Rehabil, 34:2,* 1968.

Krusen, Frank H., Kottke, Frederic, and Ellwood, Paul M. (Eds.): *Handbook of Physical Medicine and Rehabilitation.* Philadelphia, W. B. Saunders, 1966.

Maslow, Abraham H.: *Motivation and Personality,* 2d ed. New York, Harper & Row, 1970.

Neff, Walter: *Work and Human Behavior.* New York, Atherton Press, 1968.

Savine, Mike, Belchick, Jerry, and Brean, Edna: *Rehabilitation Record.* Washington, U. S. Department of Health, Education, and Welfare, 1971.

Wax, John: The inner life, a new dimension of rehabilitation. *J Rehabil, 38:6,* 1972.

CHAPTER 13

THE ADMINISTRATION OF HOMEBOUND REHABILITATION PROGRAMS

HERBERT RUSALEM and MILTON COHEN

MORE THAN TWO MILLION Americans are so physically, intellectually, or emotionally limited that they cannot regularly participate in educational, vocational, and social activities in the community with the transportation resources that are normally available to them. The Programmatic Research Project on the Rehabilitation of Homebound Persons (Rusalem, 1972) conducted by Federation of the Handicapped with the support of the Social and Rehabilitation Service clearly demonstrated two overreaching facts about this vast group:

1. Fewer than 5 percent of the homebound who can benefit from rehabilitation services are receiving such services.
2. Those who are receiving services benefit substantially from them and, in the process, require no major alterations in current rehabilitation practices to do so.

The central conclusion derived from seven years of research in this project is that rehabilitation agency administrators constitute the single most impermeable barrier to independent living for homebound persons. This barrier is even greater in its effect upon homebound persons than the severity of their disabilities, the apathy of the community, and the expected difficulties that are encountered in delivering service to this group. Indeed, once an administrator decides that he has a responsibility for, and a commitment to, the rehabilitation of homebound persons, forces are set in motion which almost immediately bring the rehabilitation of this group out of the realm of the impossible into the realm of the practical.

The conclusive evidence for this statement was derived from an intensive field study of fifty agencies offering differentiated homebound rehabilitation services. These agencies come in all sizes, shapes, and types; they cover the total spectrum of rehabilitation facilities in the United States, with only one major factor in common; they serve homebound people. When a comparison was drawn between these fifty agencies and fifty others that do not work with homebound persons, only one variable differentiated the two categories. Contrary to expectations, this variable was not fiscal status, the level of sophistication of the staff or the administration, the philosophy of the agency, the community in which it is located, its place in the community, nor the other types of rehabilitation programs which it offers. The one thing that counted was an administrator who saw service to the homebound as the mission of his organization and who felt a personal commitment to see to it that this mission was fulfilled.

Given this initial critical variable, all other obstacles to homebound rehabilitation programming were overcome, and the obstacles are numerous. As demonstrated by the very ordinary agencies that are now regularly serving homebound clients without facing impending bankruptcy or disruption to their other programs, the problems are manageable. This chapter will suggest some of the techniques that administrators are using in everyday practice to cope with these problems. As a preliminary step, however, it is advisable to buttress the argument that common garden-variety administrative procedures do succeed in making the rehabilitation of homebound persons a feasible enterprise for many facilities.

Some of the most persuasive data on this point emerged from the handful of state rehabilitation agencies that offer defined homebound rehabilitation services. The prototype of all succeeding programs was developed during the years of the Great Depression of the thirties by courageous and far-seeing rehabilitation administrators in the State of Wisconsin. Stirred by the desperate situation of the homebound in that state and moved by a vision that they could be assisted, these administrators established the Wisconsin Homecrafters, a program that continues today to be one of the outstanding efforts of its type in the world. Interestingly, despite evidence of well over thirty years of experience in this program, there still are some administrators of state rehabilitation agencies who believe that it cannot or should not be done.

Along with a few other states, New York currently offers a vigorous and dynamic homebound rehabilitation program that traces its roots back more than twenty years. In assessing this experience, it is well to keep in mind that the New York State Office of Vocational Rehabilitation (OVR) conforms closely to the typical state rehabilitation agency. It has similar struggles in funding its program properly; it has the customary personnel recruitment and training problems; it is coping with a vastly increased caseload of more complex rehabilitation problems, and it is affected by larger social and political movements in the state and federal government, not all of which are consistently favorable to rehabilitation. In short, it has nothing special going for it. On the contrary, those associated with the agency might take the position that New York State has more than its share of rehabilitation problems. Despite this, the New York State Office of Vocational Rehabilitation rehabilitates hundreds of homebound persons every year without special grants or other resources and without major alterations in the basic state rehabilitation agency structure and process. Indeed, the rehabilitation of the homebound has become so commonplace at this agency that it is almost taken for granted as much as the rehabilitation of leg amputees, the educable mentally retarded, or the cardiac.

How does New York do it? In the early 1950's, an OVR administrator became concerned about homebound citizens in New York and resolved that steps should be taken to bring these people under his agency's service umbrella. Within a period of months, it was found that not only was the goal feasible, but it generated important benefits for the community and the agency as well. Among these are a reduction in the need for public assistance among members of the caseload, reduced economic and social pressure on the family, prevention of institutionalization, increases in income and other tax payments by these clients, and general enrichment of the community.

An intensive investigation by the Programmatic Research Project of New York's OVR Homebound Rehabilitation experience clearly indicated the following:

1. The rate of rehabilitation case closures achieved with homebound clients is comparable to that found in other OVR severe disability caseloads.

2. The average cost of rehabilitating homebound people is no more than $200 above the national average cost per rehabilitation closure. More important, this average cost was less than that of certain other disability groups that have been served by rehabilitation agencies for many decades, including the totally blind, the paraplegic, the disabled college student, and the double amputee.

3. The results of the New York State experience cannot be attributed to OVR cooperation with any single specialized agency. In this instance, only 25 percent of the homebound cases served were helped with the cooperation of Federation of the Handicapped which does have special homebound rehabilitation resources. In actual practice, more than twenty-five different community agencies actually participated in joint OVR programming for the homebound in a typical year.

4. Although the most evident advance made by these homebound clients was in relation to income, substantial other gains were observed, including improvement in family and institutional acceptance and adjustment, higher levels of self-care, enhanced intellectual and cognitive functioning, heightened self-awareness and self-regard, and greater involvement in community, home, and leisure activities. In almost every respect, these homebound persons were motivated to use the program effectively and constituted a fairly easy group with which to work.

5. Although considerable imagination, creativity, and involvement are required in homebound rehabilitation, unselected counselors on a state agency staff can function satisfactorily with homebound clients if properly oriented and trained. In practice, New York OVR assigns its counselors to homebound service without regard to their particular excellence

or special attributes. While some are better than others in serving the homebound, this is the case in regard to counselors working with any other caseload.

6. The rehabilitation outcomes of the New York State OVR Homebound Program tend to be long-term in nature. Follow-up studies conducted by the Programmatic Research Project of agency homebound cases revealed that most homebound clients retain their newly acquired jobs for years, even decades.

7. Perhaps, the most striking finding of all in this study was that some 20 percent of the homebound cases served by the New York State OVR, became non-homebound in the course of rehabilitation. This was accomplished by the State Agency Counselors through physical and emotional restoration, lessening the impact of architectural barriers, and counseling and environmental adjustments that reduced psychosocial barriers to community participation.

8. Finally, it was found that the growth impetus of this homebound rehabilitation program has not lessened over the years. On the contrary, the homebound caseload is still expanding, rehabilitation techniques are becoming evermore sophisticated, and cooperating community agencies are becoming more numerous and effective.

The central conclusion that can be drawn from the successful New York State OVR experience is that any of the other State Rehabilitation Agencies that choose to do so can follow this model and, probably, can achieve similar outcomes. Indeed, several other states have already followed New York State and others are on the verge of doing so. The key is whether a State Agency administration has the will. Similarly, among voluntary rehabilitation agencies, such organizations as Federation of the Handicapped, the Iowa Easter Seal Society, the Missouri Easter Seal Society, the Texas Institute of Research and Rehabilitation, and many others are finding day after day that homebound rehabilitation is practical and that administrative resolve and resourcefulness are the mainsprings of service action for this group.

More than anything else, rehabilitation administrators need information about the organization and operation of homebound rehabilitation programs so that their anxiety about such programs can interact with established facts. Until relatively recently, such information was virtually unavailable. In a comprehensive review of the homebound rehabilitation literature not too many years ago, Rusalem (1967) found few references that offered practical assistance to administrators and practitioners. Today, factual materials, while not exactly abundant, are increasingly available from a growing number of sources to support the belief that homebound rehabilitation is viable in everyday agency practice. Some of this information will be presented later in this chapter. Before turning to it, however, it is important to examine still another major roadblock to program development in this area.

Among the rationalizations most frequently used to justify rehabilitation agency inaction on behalf of the homebound is the often repeated statement that the homebound have a low service priority. In these instances, priorities are used as an apparently socially acceptable explanation of administrative avoidance of one of the largest groups of disabled persons in the United States. In part, it is this misuse of existing priorities that throws the whole priority system into sharp relief. For example, recently established high priority groups have included the severely disabled, the institutionalized, the socially disadvantaged, the welfare client, and the social security recipient. In practice, homebound persons constitute a sizeable subgroup in each category, and, consequently, merit first-order attention rather than exclusion from rehabilitation service. Indeed, they form a disproportionately high percentage of public assistance clients, social security disability recipients, and institutionalized persons. Yet, the neglect of the homebound is so shocking that Congress felt it necessary to stipulate in the Rehabilitation Act of 1973 that priority in service now should officially be given to the severely disabled (including the homebound). This Congressional action is in response to the fact that some state and local agency administrators systematically exclude homebound citizens from the benefits of rehabilitation.

It is probable that the whole priority system has damaged thousands of homebound persons. Fortunately or unfortunately, rehabilitation priorities are made by men and women who are as fallible as the rest of us. They bring to the priority-setting process their own biases and predilections and are influenced by compelling political and social pressures to make expedient judgments. Consequently, they are no more in a position to play God with people's lives than anyone else. Unwarranted delay of the initiation of rehabilitation services to eligible and feasible homebound persons or exclusion therefrom undermines the whole rehabilitation system. Historically, the overarching thrust of rehabilitation has been to eradicate discrimination against the handicapped. Paradoxically, rehabilitation priorities constitute discrimination in its most pernicious form. Unfortunately, discrimination by priorities is practiced by those who are quick to decry it in employers and other gatekeepers of our society. A more acceptable concept is that if a person meets the eligibility requirements for any public or voluntary program, disqualification of that person on the basis of fallible and arbitrary priority rankings probably constitutes an infringement on the rights of that person to equal protection of the law. If such discrimination against the homebound (or any other rehabilitation group) continues, it will almost certainly be challenged in the courts. The national Congress or our state legislatures are legally constrained in their enactments by the equal protection clause of the American Constitution. Government bureaucrats and agency administrators and practitioners are no more immune from this provision in implementing rehabilitation programs than the legislators who create them. The growing advocacy movement, on behalf of the severely disabled, will become increasingly reluctant to permit the human rights of homebound persons to be abridged by arbitrary procedures and judgments.

The Home as a Rehabilitation Facility

An intensive investigation of twenty currently viable homebound rehabilitation programs (Rusalem, 1972) revealed that such programs rely heavily upon sound general administrative principles that apply to all organizational structures. In this con-

text, viable homebound rehabilitation programs are characterized by well-designed fiscal controls, economical use of personnel
and other resources, direct accountability from staff members,
wide usage of techniques that benefit the maximum number of
homebound persons at moderate cost, maintenance of parsimonious transportation arrangements and schedules, reliance upon
direct lines of command, the adoption of sound cost accounting
principles, effective production management, and the extensive
use of community and family aids and resources. Beyond this
generalization, there is one vital factor that makes a homebound
program administratively unique and that is that the program
is conducted primarily in the homes of severely disabled persons
rather than in central or satellite locations. Thus, in effect, there
are as many rehabilitation facilities, workshops, or work activities centers to administer in such a program as there are homebound persons in the caseload. This proliferation of locations
is a sufficient challenge unto itself to the rehabilitation administrators, but the wide diffusion of service sites is only one aspect
of the administrator's problem.

Beyond decentralization, the central problem of administering
a homebound program is the nature of the home as a rehabilitation facility. It is the home ecology that complicates further
an already involved rehabilitation facilities administration problem. The home ecology introduced the following special administrative complications into facilities management:

Accessibility

Instead of relatively easily managed central sites, homebound
clients' homes are distributed over a broad geographical area extending many miles beyond the agency's headquarters and even its
outreach stations. Although telephone communication is readily
established with these home sites (wherever a telephone is available in the client's home), face-to-face communication and the
pick-up and delivery of materials requires a transportation network of one kind or another. It is axiomatic in this field that
transportation constitutes the most pervasive barrier to homebound persons and concurrently, the most difficult and costly administrative problem to manage.

Inappropriateness of the Home

The design of rehabilitation facilities has become much more of a science in the past decade. In planning the establishment or the renovation of such physical quarters, specialized skills, understandings, and know-how are essential because it is evident that severely disabled persons require types of physical space and equipment that extend well beyond those found in industry or even in other community agencies. Yet, confronted by very limited homebound clients, a homebound rehabilitation program is compelled to fit its program into a home setting which generally is deficient in terms of space, physical accessibility, special aids and equipment, and, not infrequently, minimum acceptable levels of sanitation, ventilation, light and comfort. In some instances, the physical ecology of the home is found to be so physically and emotionally limited that it is impossible to conduct almost any type of rehabilitation service there. Thus, even counseling services may be difficult to offer because privacy cannot be assured for interviewing. As far as a work program is concerned, a home setting almost always leaves much to be desired.

Impact of Ongoing Relationships

Every home is an arena in which complex and troublesome interpersonal relationships are played out. In some instances, these relationships facilitate the homebound rehabilitation program. Unfortunately, in most cases, they do not. Every family uses the homebound person in its own way to fulfill its own ends. In all too many cases, these responses benefit non-disabled family members but not the homebound person. Thus, family overprotection, overt and more subtle rejection, infantilization, or open aggression swirl about the client and the rehabilitation worker as they attempt to work through critical disability problems. In a central facility, although the client does not fully escape the enervating effects of these relationships, at least he has counteracting experiences while he is in the special center environment. Often, these center experiences provide an effective immunization of the disabled person against family shelter and offers him an anchor upon which to establish more realistic and healthy self-perceptions. In the home, there is no such counter-balance. Both the client and the worker are enmeshed in emotionally charged situations over which they have little control and which well may vitiate the rehabilitation services delivered to the severely disabled person.

Family or Community Interference

Family members, neighbors, and even community agency staff members may interject themselves into various aspects of home-bound rehabilitation. Such interjection ranges from outsiders monopolizing the worker's attention when he visits the home, thus depriving the client of a vitally needed professional time, to others doing the client's assigned remunerative homework for him. Since the rehabilitation worker is present in the home only occasionally and, then for very brief periods of time, agency control of local interferences is virtually impossible. Such interferences often are well-meaning, but they sometimes mask hostile impulses and aggression toward the severely handicapped person. The administrative challenge is to find means of preventing or limiting such damaging interventions and converting the significant others in the home into contributing members of the rehabilitation service team.

The Isolation Component

Interaction with peers is one of the principal dynamics of a rehabilitation facility program. Through getting feedback from other disabled persons and through observing their rehabilitation struggles and successes, many rehabilitation clients are stimulated to work on their own problems and to seek their own solutions. Indeed some rehabilitation facilities use successful rehabilitation clients as role-models for newer clients. In this manner, fantasy elements in the self-concept, unreal expectations, and unwarranted despair are all reality-tested with one's contemporaries. In the home, however, the severely disabled client has few opportunities to reality-test his notions about himself and others and cannot readily share his rehabilitation experience with other disabled persons who may give him a quality of support and understanding that professional workers cannot provide. Thus, one of the critical variables in rehabilitation service, that of group experiences, is absent in the home milieu.

Dependency Reinforcement in the Home

Most rehabilitation facilities consciously develop therapeutic environments which systematically reinforce personal, social, and vocational autonomy. Thus, the agency's physical setting, the type of supervision offered, and the counseling approaches, reward systems, and reliance upon individual decision-making all contribute to the process of gradually enhancing client independence. On the other hand, such a therapeutic environment is infinitely more difficult to create in the home. Because of this, many relationships, physical features, family, activities and interpersonal attitudes in the home attenuate rather than expand personal self-direction. Not infrequently, these factors engender so much conflict on the part of the homebound client that he becomes paralyzed, being unable to follow-through on his rehabilitation plan while, simultaneously, feeling some need to become more autonomous. The challenge to the administrator of this conflict and the causal reinforcement of dependency in the family is to find means of introducing program components into the home that foster greater client independence and self-sustenance in the face of these debilitative elements.

The Customary Function of the Home

Many years ago, the home was a focus for family educational and vocational activity and a place where a person's physical and mental health problems could receive proper care. In those days of extended family nurturance, many jobs were performed in or near the home and relatively few persons entered long-term hospitals and institutions. Home was where the action was, where essential life functions were carried on and where family members served each other in times of need. Today's nuclear family undertakes quite different functions. Although it still provides some emotional and social support and a certain amount of social activity, it is, in many cases, only a kinship dormitory where food and clothing are provided by a breadwinner and some socialized behaviors are taught by example and direct instruction. In such a setting, home rehabilitation and employment may be intrusive and even unwelcome. Thus, the introduction of rehabilitation and work interventions into a severely disabled person's home can upset established routines and family concepts and arouse anxiety and uneasiness. Indeed, the administration of a homebound rehabilitation program often requires providing for family counseling that, hopefully, will minimize such reactions. Otherwise, the home becomes an antagonistic rather than a cooperative rehabilitation factor.

Psychological Response of the Professional Worker

In its least virulent form, a negative response to homeboundedness on the part of the professional worker can be an ideological barrier. Thus, the worker may have learned from leadership personnel and more experienced contemporaries that rehabilitation in the home, if it occurs at all, does so with infinite difficulty and frustration. In this framework, he interjects into his professional thinking the mythology that the home of a disabled person is an impossible rehabilitation setting. This mythology tenaciously supports the widespread belief that rehabilitation cannot happen there. Not infrequently, this ideology is cloaked with pious disclaimers of rejection of homebound clients and voluble protestation of belief in homebound rehabilitation programs. In fact, persuasive rationales often are offered by such workers to forestall their own anxiety and guilt. These rationales tend to be phrased in terms of presumed costs, inaccessibility of clients, insuperable service problems, and, now and then, by sonorous pontifications that no disabled persons live in a particular jurisdiction or that the few who do live there are too aged, too feeble, or too poorly motivated to qualify for rehabilitation service. Since these rationales lack validity, there is some suspicion that a proportion of rehabilitation workers are emotionally troubled by the homebound condition and, rather than facing these feelings directly, some of them build a web of rationalizations for their inaction and avoidance. Just as certain disabilities arouse distress in some rehabilitation workers, so does homeboundedness trouble some of our colleagues. However innocent or even unconscious that these feelings may be, their net effect is to exclude homebound persons from the rehabilitation services that they need.

If a homebound rehabilitation program is to be effective, the rehabilitation administrator will be required to manifest all the sound professional behaviors that mark good facility administration. In general, however, in addition to providing leadership to the staff, the clients, and the community, setting a role-model for all concerned by reason of his commitment to the homebound group, and orchestrating all program and management elements into an efficient approach to the problems of the homebound group, the rehabilitation administrator will have to find means of coping with the eight attributes of a home rehabilitation setting noted briefly above. He will have to find some way of managing these factors so that homebound rehabilitation becomes a feasible enterprise at this agency. Listed below are a few of the approaches used by successful homebound programs in handling such troublesome elements. However, it should be kept in mind that no two agency situations are the same and that the solutions of one are not necessarily applicable to others.

I. Administration of Accessibility Services

Administrators of homebound rehabilitation programs have solved accessibility problems through both bringing the homebound client to the service and bringing the service to the home.

A. *Bringing the Client to the Service*

When physical movement of a homebound client to the rehabilitation facility is medically approved, logistically possible, and administratively economical, it has the irrefutable advantage of revising the homebound person's status so that he becomes a mobile rehabilitation client. This opens vast new rehabilitation opportunities for him that will be beyond his reach as long as he remains homebound.

Such an approach is most feasible in a compact geographical area where appropriate transportation facilities can be arranged and when clients are ready, willing, and able to leave their homes. Among the techniques used to bring such clients to the service facility are:

1. Agency-operated minibuses or other special agency-operated transportation facilities that pick up homebound clients on a regular basis.
2. The use of volunteer drivers. Although this is the most economical approach, it is exceedingly difficult to maintain on an ongoing scheduled basis.
3. Taxicabs, private contract drivers, and on-call buses.
4. Movement of the client into a residence that is far closer to the rehabilitation facility than his regular residence.
5. Developing foster or group home programs that bring the client into residences near the rehabilitation facility.
6. Conducting evaluation and training activities in a summer or year-round camp environment.
7. Housing clients in an intermediate care or long-term illness facility near the rehabilitation agency.
8. Developing car pools staffed by agency personnel and/or more mobile clients.
9. Having the client participate regularly in agency-sponsored conference telephone calls that provide him with group experiences and group supervision.
10. Developing a paid core of poverty-area residents who, when provided with vehicles, assume responsibility for transporting homebound persons.

B. *Bringing the Service to the Client*

Very severe physical, intellectual, and emotional conditions, geographic inaccessibility, lack of emotional readiness to disengage oneself from the home situation, lack of transportation resources, and extreme family resistance may prevent regular attendance of the homebound client at central or outreach rehabilitation facilities. In these instances (perhaps, while efforts are being made to prepare the client as soon as possible to transfer into the established local facility), services will be brought to the client. These services usually include intake and evaluation, counseling, family guidance, socialization, personal adjustment and skills training, home employment, follow-up, and health care. Obviously, services delivered to the home are generally less comprehensive and systematic than in a rehabilitation facility but, still, infinitely superior to no service at all.

Among the techniques that have been used administratively to manage problems in this area have been:

1. The use of agency-owned or rented vehicles to transport agency staff members to clients' homes.
2. The use of public transportation to bring agency personnel, goods, and services to the home. This approach has value in a limited number of cases in which public transportation is adequate and personnel time loss in traveling is not a crucial factor.
3. The use of messengers (such as mentally retarded clients) to deliver raw materials and pick up finished products from the client's residence.
4. The employment of part-time local aides (perhaps qualified housewives) to bring goods and services to the homebound individual.
5. Using agency vehicles stationed at local "drops" or outreach stations that are closer to client's home than is the central agency facility.
6. Using United Parcel Service, Greyhound and Trailways Buses, and other public carriers to pick up and deliver merchandise near the client's home.
7. Using volunteer drivers to make deliveries.
8. Contracting with local trucking firms to make pickups and deliveries.
9. Having family members of the client take responsibility for merchandise deliveries.
10. Using trained and supervised poverty program partic-

ipant as homebound aides to bring both merchandise and services to the homebound individual (typified by the well-established PATH—Personal Aides to the Homebound—Program conducted by Federation of the Handicapped).

II. Administrative Steps to Counteract Limitations in the Home Setting

The initial step in this area is almost always a survey of the client's home to ascertain the availability of suitable resources and the presence of persistent problems, including family attitudes, financial problems, transportation, readiness of neighbors to cooperate, architectural barriers, possible work space, recreation facilities, sanitation, ventilation, light, and linkages between the home and the church, local health facilities, and social and fraternal organizations. Invariably, such a survey indicates that there are shortcomings as well as strengths in the home situation. The strengths are taken into account in planning home-based programs and the limitations become the subject of agency-initiated interventions. Throughout this procedure, every effort is made to alter the home both physically and psychosocially to expedite the rehabilitation of the homebound persons. Agencies have taken the following steps to strengthen the home environment:

A. Family counseling around steps that can be taken to provide a healthier emotional climate for the homebound person.

B. Planning physical modifications in space, attractiveness, sanitation, lighting, and ventilation that will render the client more efficient and more comfortable.

C. Working with hospitals, health centers, physicians, and organizations to create a more healthful environment for the client.

D. Requesting assistance from a home economics specialist in redesigning home facilities and home organization so that the client can become as self-sufficient as possible in such activities as self-care, mobility in and out of the home, and the use of home resources.

E. Assessing the possible impact upon the client's family of introducing remunerative work in the home and easing this impact, when necessary, by providing counseling and reassurance and by encouraging family participation in all phases of rehabilitation planning.

F. Working with welfare and other public and voluntary support agencies to equip the home with various appliances and devices that will foster client independence.

G. Arranging for work tables, chairs, lamps, machines, and equipment needed to maximize client efficiency.

H. Developing clean-up procedures for the client and his family so that the space used for remunerative work can be converted to other family purposes when desired.

I. Evolving a suitable procedure for storing raw materials and finished products in the home so that the regular flow of family life is not disrupted.

J. Informing the family of the rigid provisions of national, state, and local laws relating to homework and noting that violations of these provisions can result in discontinuance of all homework activity.

Obviously, no amount of environmental modification will make a client's home equivalent to a rehabilitation facility. At best, even a modified home milieu will contain numerous flaws and barriers but then the goal is not perfection. If the home can be made even moderately more suitable for rehabilitation activities despite residual limitation, this will be a major contribution to the client's rehabilitation. Administrators in the homebound rehabilitation area should insist that their staffs make every possible move toward enriching the home environment but only after it has been clearly and unequivocally determined that rehabilitation in the home is the only viable rehabilitation alternative at the moment.

III. Managing the Program's Impact on Ongoing Relationships

The introduction of homework into a homebound person's residence can be perceived by some family members as an invasion of private life-space. Others may view it as an attempt to wean the homebound person away from his family or as a means of reducing his need to lean on family members. In some situations, families resent homework because it may delay planned institutionalized or placement of the homebound person in some other out-of-home situation. In actual service experience, a whole gamut of family reactions may be expected to homebound rehabilitation efforts because such efforts upset the current balance of interpersonal forces in the home and, however difficult the current situation is, the status quo may be less threatening than the consequences that may follow homebound rehabilitation. Agencies serving homebound persons have dealt with these feelings in a number of ways:

A. Family members are involved in rehabilitation planning for the homebound client from the onset of service.

B. The family unit is perceived by the rehabilitation worker as the real client in the situation and rehabilitation or equivalent services are made available to all members of the group.

C. Rehabilitation plans are implemented very gradually so that change does not occur too precipitously in the rehabilitation process.

D. Family members are assigned paraprofessional roles in the rehabilitation program, such as serving as assistant trainers, inspectors of finished work, and academic and vocational tutors.

E. Family counseling agencies in the community are invited to participate in the rehabilitation program established for a family unit.

F. Family counseling, rather than individual counseling, is made the fulcrum of the rehabilitation effort.

G. Carefully conducted family planning helps to set space and activity limits for the client's remunerative homework experiences.

In brief, although family participation is important in all rehabilitation programming, it is even more critical in the rehabilitation of homebound persons and, thus, it should be accorded special administrative consideration in formulating and implementing rehabilitation programming for this client group.

IV. Family or Community Interference

The entry of the rehabilitation worker into a homebound individual's home can be perceived as a major social event or, conversely, as a major invasion of family privacy. At either end of this scale or at any point in between, family and community members may behave in ways that interfere with the delivery of rehabilitation service. For example, family members may overwhelm the agency worker with hospitality, prevent the client from speaking for himself, or instruct the agency worker how to do his job, or engage in a variety of other activities that deter client progress. Even more serious are the attempts of some family members to discourage the client from participating in rehabilitation activities, underscoring the hopelessness of the proposed rehabilitation efforts. Unless such behaviors can be prevented or remediated without delay, rehabilitation progress may be slow or nonexistent. Agencies offering homebound rehabilitation services manage these problems by:

A. Family involvement and counseling as noted in Section III above.

B. Offering as many rehabilitation services as possible outside the home.

C. Counseling the client concerning these interfering behaviors hopefully encouraging him to accept and use the preferred service despite others' negative views.

D. Enlisting the support and help of family physicians, visiting nurses, and other professional individuals who concurrently are serving the homebound person and his family.

E. Setting limits with the family and the neighbors, indicating for them and the client the conditions under which service can be rendered and requiring all concerned to meet these standards for the sake of the client's ultimate rehabilitation.

F. If all else fails, discussing with the client the desirability and feasibility of relocating in a foster home or some other type of community residence.

Deterrent family behaviors are difficult to control because they are firmly rooted in people's attitudinal structures. The most favorable administrative step that can be taken to forestall or minimize such behaviors is for administration to spell out clearly to the family, the client, and the worker the conditions under which homebound rehabilitation service will be delivered. If these conditions are violated, efforts should be made through counseling, casework, and other interventions to remedy the situation. Failing that, all participants should be made aware of the consequences of continued deterrent responses and, if necessary, rehabilitation service may be deferred until proper conditions for its delivery are established.

V. The Isolation Component

Homebound people report that one of the most painful sequelae of homeboundedness is the monotony and boredom that fills their days. Many of these individuals turn on the television early in the day and separate themselves from it only for short periods of time until retiring in the evening. Almost invariably there just isn't enough for homebound people to do in the home. Empty hour follows empty hour and almost any break in the deadening routine is welcomed. The personal dread and despair that eventuates is not the only or even the most serious consequence of this situation. The fact is that deprivation of essential life stimuli, including interactions with others, engagement in useful and productive activity, and variation in daily routines over the long-run, all reduce the responsivity, alertness, and motivation of the homebound individual. In time, this may result in cumulative disengagement from the environment and a cycle of progressive voluntary isolations that can lead to prolonged emotional problems and ultimate institutionalization. Agencies serving the homebound use the following means to work with these isolation problems.

A. If at all possible, the individual is taken out of the home, even if once a week.

B. Volunteer or paid workers are regularly assigned to visit the client, provide companionship to him, share experiences with him, engage in recreation activities, and bring to him news of the outside world.

C. Talking books or records and cassettes are provided the homebound person so that he can benefit from the stimulation of the printed word as it appears in books, magazines, and other forms of communication.

D. If the homebound person is academically inclined, arrangements are made for him to take recorded or correspondence courses on a high school equivalency and adult education level.

E. The homebound person is involved in conference telephone discussion groups, adult courses, and group social conversations following the innovative model pioneered by Federation of the Handicapped.

F. Community volunteers, such as members of a high school students' homebound service corps are assigned to visit homebound persons and engage them in a variety of activities.

G. Homebound persons in a particular neighborhood are brought together in an outreach location, sometimes in the home of one of the group members, where informal social and educational programming can be conducted.

H. Home-to-agency telephone service (comparable to home-to-school programs) are set up in which homebound persons participate in group programs conducted from agency premises through telephonic means.

I. Special vehicles are used to take homebound persons on trips in the community or, as in the case of Federation of the Handicapped, even on international tours.

J. Special transportation is arranged on an occasional basis to bring homebound persons to special community or agency social or educational events.

In some instances administrative provisions are made only for remunerative work. Although such programs are invaluable, they fill only part of the psychosocial needs of homebound individuals. Unless concomitant socialization programs are developed to reduce isolation, the psychosexual results of homework may be limited, indeed.

VI. Dependency Reinforcement in the Home

The central goal of homebound rehabilitation is the enhancement of client independence but the central goal of the client's family may be something else. Early in the homebound experience, the client has to establish a balance between his concurrent needs for both independence and dependence. Although this is a lifelong struggle for all of us, homebound individuals face many special in-home reinforcements, because of the dependency implied in their family status. Family and friends often react to the homebound person in ways that reward his conformance to the helplessness stereotype that most people maintain of homebound people.

Awash in pity, guilt, and oversolicitousness, they make it easy and pleasant to be dependent. Into this situation in which the dependence of the homebound person may be enshrined and almost worshipped comes the rehabilitation worker advocating greater independence. Understandably, universal joy and relief do not always accompany his offers of a better life for the disabled person. Given the family and community resistances that are likely to be stirred up by rehabilitation efforts, many homebound rehabilitation plans have been sabotaged by family appeals to clients' dependency needs. Agencies serving the homebound have attempted to cope with these behaviors through the following means:

A. If it can be arranged, some or all of the rehabilitation program is conducted outside the home.

B. Family and client counseling are made essential components of the rehabilitation experience.

C. The rehabilitation worker consistently serves as a positive reinforcer of client behaviors that augur greater independence.

D. In treating the homebound client with respect and in requiring him to make his own decisions, the rehabilitation worker helps him to gain a new percept of himself as a person and sets a desirable role model for family members and others who relate to the client.

E. A specialist in self-care, life-skills, and/or home economics is assigned to train the homebound person to perform as many daily tasks for himself as possible. These training activities are conducted with the approval and cooperation of medical and other health care personnel and have as their goal the demonstration of client capacities to do more for himself.

F. Family members and volunteers are trained in methods of fostering client independence.

G. Rehabilitation activities are introduced to the client in graduated sequences of small steps which virtually assure mastery of the tasks to be performed. This success experience is used as a positive reinforcer of client feeling of self-worth and self-reliance.

H. If the client enters a remunerative homework program, he is helped to use his earnings in a manner best calculated to improve his status in the home. For example, his contributions to the support of the household, however moderate they may be, are useful as a lever in gaining respect from others, such as granting the homebound individual a role in family decision-making processes.

Independence is such a critical variable in determining whether a homebound rehabilitation program will be successful that specific administrative planning for services in this area is essential.

VII. The Customary Function of the Home

The central problem in this regard occurs when remunerative homework is thought by the family to be incompatible with a home situation and an infringement on their territoriality.

Understandably averse to having home space which they use for the other purposes allotted to work benches and tables, they react negatively to the use of closets or corners for the storage of materials; they object to the appearance of tools, equipment, and merchandise that are out in the open; they deplore the apparent or imagined dirt, disorder, and clutter that they associate with work activities. Unless these feelings can be eased, the homework program will run into continuing family opposition. Thus, agencies serving the homebound use one or more of the following interventions to make homework more acceptable:

A. Homework items are kept as small, light, and unobtrusive as possible.

B. Wherever feasible, homework equipment is made portable and convertible. Preferably, work benches, chairs, and other equipment can be folded into compact packages and stored out of sight with little effort.

C. The client is taught to be orderly, neat, and systematic in his work. He is instructed how to avoid clutter and work residuals when he finishes his daily job activities by cleaning up his work space thoroughly even though this takes additional time and effort.

D. Joint planning with the family is conducted to select a functional work space in the home that will cause the least family disruption and distaste.

E. The homebound program staff works with the client and the family to engineer and design the work space so that it is as attractive and functional as possible.

F. As early as possible, family members are given an opportunity to discuss their feelings about the introduction of work tasks and materials into the home.

G. New work tasks are assigned to the homebound client only after they have been demonstrated to, and approved by, family members.

H. Regular pickup and delivery schedules are maintained

by the agency, and these do not allow an excessive quantity of work materials or finished products to accumulate in the home.

I. Periodic spot inspections of the homework area are conducted by the agency to ascertain if the client is functioning in the manner in which he was trained and currently is maintaining the work area at a level that is tolerable to the family.

J. Insofar as possible, noisy, unsightly, and disturbing tools and equipment are avoided.

In addition to helping family members to deal with their feelings about remunerative homework, every administrative effort should be made to reduce the potency of work stimuli for generating family displeasure and resistance. Unless this is done, the family may discourage the homebound individual from participating in the program, causing premature withdrawal from the service and consequent unsuccessful case closure.

VIII. Administrative Considerations Relating to Psychological Responses of the Professional Worker

Some administrators and clinicians offer very limited services to homebound persons. The reasons they offer for this are less than convincing in the light of current knowledge and experience. Undoubtedly, different clusters of personal and professional dynamics enter into this attitude among different administrators and workers. Among those that were identified by the Programmatic Research Project on the Rehabilitation of the Homebound Persons were personal anxiety in the presence of homeboundedness, the desire to play a stationary office-based (as opposed to an active field) role in one's professional life, the presumed difficulty of rehabilitating homebound clients, lack of proper reward and reinforcement systems for serving the homebound, lack of previous experience in serving the homebound, fear of failure, and the inexorable pressures of the numbers game in which the box score of cases closed successfully is more important than quality of performance.

Since the acceptance, energy, creativity, and warmth of the worker is crucial in the rehabilitation of homebound persons, the following administrative provisions have been made by agencies serving homebound individuals:

A. Only those rehabilitation workers who have demonstrated an affinity for homebound clients are assigned to these clients.

B. A special homebound service unit is established which specializes in working with severely disabled persons confined to their homes.

C. Agency leadership overtly and forcefully supports the homebound rehabilitation program and sets a model for the agency staff in unequivocally advocating the rights of homebound people.

D. Special rewards are offered to rehabilitation workers who serve the severely disabled.

E. Through supervision, reluctant and recalcitrant workers are helped to understand their feelings about the homebound and are given opportunities to work through their problems in delivering rehabilitation service to them.

F. Intensive training in the special techniques of serving homebound persons is provided to professional and nonprofessional workers throughout the agency.

G. Every agency worker and supervisor who is not emotionally threatened by the prospect is required to carry some homebound cases so that he can test his concepts about the group against the realities of everyday service.

H. Group sessions or *retreats* are conducted (often with the help of group dynamics specialists) at which staff members are encouraged to examine their feelings about homebound persons.

Whenever the above interventions fail to augment staff acceptance and performance in relation to homebound clients, consideration should be given to the reassignment of personnel to other caseloads and to the possibility of disengaging the worker from service to the severely disabled.

Selecting an Administrative Route to
Homebound Programming

From an administrative viewpoint, it is wise to launch home-bound rehabilitation programming on a small (even a pilot) scale using an initial tested model. Each of the following approaches has been used by one or more public and voluntary agencies as their preferred route to homebound programming. The selection of a model depends upon local needs, resources, and philosophies. None is intrinsically superior to the others, but some are more appropriate than others for specified local conditions. The decision about which route a community should follow is one that can only be made by the agencies and groups concerned. Therefore, the material presented below is not meant to be prescriptive. On the contrary, it is merely a catalogue of presently-used homebound rehabilitation program models that may indicate to program planners the wide range of approaches now being used in serving this population.

The Health Care Model

This model was created in response to the finding that many homebound persons do not have ready access to medical, dental, nursing, physical and occupational therapy, and related health services. The consequences of this deprivation is the persistence and exacerbation of health conditions that generate and, in some cases, prolong homeboundedness. The central thrust of this model is to bring health personnel into the home through itinerant worker arrangements, mobile units, or local outreach stations.

As a result of improved health service delivery, some home-bound persons have been rendered non-homebound and others have been helped to lead more comfortable and useful lives in the home and the community.

The Home Economics Model

Pioneered by Dr. Lois Schwab at the University of Nebraska and other home economics specialists, this approach views the home as a modifiable home life ecology that can be enriched immeasurably for the homebound person. The core goal is the improvement of the homebound individual's efficiency in his residence, not merely to augment the quality of living in the home, but wherever possible, to enable the homebound person to be less homebound and more active in his community. Although home economists play a leading role in this service pattern, they do so in the framework of an interdisciplinary team that takes a holistic view of the homebound individual and his problems.

The Recreation Model

This approach focuses upon the evident social deprivation suffered by many homebound persons and attempts to foster happier and more useful living by training the person in leisure pursuits, providing recreational counseling, and involving him in carefully structured recreational activities. All these efforts are designed to make the world a more interesting place for the client, but equally important, long-range objectives are pursued in the areas of self-care, independence, emotional stability, interpersonal relationships, and ties to the community.

The Home Aid Model

Home aid programming recognizes the inability of many homebound persons to be fully self-sufficient in self-care and home management, even with training. For such persons, institutionalization often is an imminent and dreaded possibility. In order to forestall entry into congregate residences and the debilitation that may result therefrom, this model shores up the person in his home, enabling him to remain there by assuring that he will receive essential personal care, live in sanitary and reasonably pleasant circumstances, be properly fed, and receive some degree of personal interest and nurturance. This service often is delivered to the homebound individual by trained paraprofessionals serving under skilled agency supervision.

The Institutional Model

The Programmatic Research Project on the Rehabilitation of Homebound Persons discovered that the negative effects of prolonged institutionalization derive not so much from congregate living under protective circumstances as upon the impoverishing nature of the man-made environment that prevails in such institutions. The institutional model accepts the inevitability of residential care, for some severely disabled persons, but not its deleterious effects. Thus, it seeks to enrich, extend, and humanize the residential milieu converting it from a stultifying, impersonal and enervating environment into a dynamic, accepting, busy, and productive place where severely limited persons may develop, enjoy life, study, and even engage in remunerative work.

The Vocational Crafts Model

In this model, homebound persons are taught to produce craft items for sale to others. Central planning, designing, instructional, and supervisory services enable homebound individuals to make and market items that attract prospective purchasers. In an era when handmade goods are rare, such craft items have special appeal to a segment of the community despite the fact that their cost may be higher than comparable machine-made products. Craft items produced in this way are marketed by a central service conducted by the agency or by the sales efforts of the homebound person, himself, perhaps in cooperation with a profit-making sales organization.

The Self-employment Model

Participants in this model are trained to conduct small business enterprises from their homes in such fields as real estate, bookkeeping, secretarial and typing services, photocopying, key-making and newspaper clipping. After being trained in a particular field, the homebound person is helped to launch his private business and, then, proceeds to develop it with continuing advice and guidance. In conducting his business, the homebound person operates just as any business entrepeneur would except for the fact that he does not routinely leave his work premises, i.e. his home, to transact his business.

The Subcontract Model

Usually associated with an ongoing sheltered workshop in the community, this model selects suitable workshop tasks for manu-

facture by homebound persons, instructs them in the performance of these tasks, provides them with raw materials, picks up
finished products, and supervises the total productive effort. In
a sense, the home becomes a sheltered workshop site which is
governed by national, state, and local wages and hours' regulations and other legal provisions, just as any workshop is so regu-
lated.

The Work Activity Model

Similar to the Subcontract Model, this approach places less
stress upon productivity, manufacturing schedules, work pressures, and rigid quality standards. On the contrary, the work activities experience in the home is perceived more as a therapeutic
than a career experience for the homebound person. In this respect, it is comparable to some recreation programs for the
homebound, except that it deals with real work tasks and a reasonably realistic work environment. Remuneration for this work
is modest, having its greatest value as a means of keeping voca-
tionally-oriented persons who cannot qualify for workshop assignments busy, interested, and involved in a work enterprise.

The Central or Outreach Work Site Model

This type of vocational programming conducts few, if any,
rehabilitation activities in the home. Instead, it makes every effort to transport homebound persons to a central or outreach rehabilitation facility or it provides a residence near such facilities.
Having brought the person to the facility, the agency then admin-
isters the homebound client's program just as it would that of any
other workshop client. The central problems in this model are developing a viable client transport system, arranging for nearby
residences for homebound clients, and fostering client willingness
and readiness to be brought closer to the facility.

The Direct Employer Contact Model

In this approach, homebound persons are evaluated and
trained by the rehabilitation agency and helped to make contact
with employers who are interested in hiring homebound workers.

The decision to hire is made by the employer and, after the rehabilitation agency assists in the initial job adjustment of the homebound worker, subsequent work experiences are shaped by negotiations between the employer and the homebound person without the direct mediation of a third party agency.

The Mixed Model

In this model, one or more of the above components are combined in a total homebound rehabilitation program. Such an arrangement, of course, multiplies both opportunities for service and administrative problems. However, it constitutes a vital development in homebound rehabilitation programming since no single program component or service model can, in and of itself, meet the needs of more than a fraction of all homebound persons. Through offering different routes to rehabilitation in a mixed model, agencies establish a situation that is more equivalent to that of other rehabilitation caseloads in that it offers options rather than a fixed unyielding stereotyped program.

The Comprehensive Model

Much more of an ideal today than a reality, this approach offers as wide a gamut of services and opportunities for homebound persons as is usually offered for other clients. Thus, it includes elements of all or many of the models noted above. In such a program, it would be possible to provide individualized rehabilitation planning for every homebound client so that his rehabilitation experiences would be custom-designed to match his needs. Although one or two agencies such as Federation of the Handicapped are moving toward that goal, its ultimate realization is far down the pike.

The models described above do not exhaust the possible approaches available for the rehabilitation of homebound persons. Indeed, new ones are already on the drawing board and should emerge into their demonstration phase during the 1970's. Suffice it to say that at this point, even if rehabilitation were to be limited to the models described above, progress in this field would cease. A few dozen rehabilitation agencies now offer one and even fewer offer two or more of these alternatives to homebound clients.

Without generating further research and demonstration findings, there is still so much to be done implementing existing findings that it would keep us busy for a long time to come. Indeed, the application of what we already know about homebound rehabilitation to actual programming will constitute a challenge for at least the next twenty to thirty years.

The Financing of Homebound Rehabilitation Programs

Although the costs of rehabilitating homebound persons are not as great as many rehabilitation administrators seem to believe, the fiscal aspects of the situation still merit extensive discussion. The most challenging fiscal condition usually arises after the rehabilitation phase of client service comes to a close. Until that time, reasonable state rehabilitation agency fees can be negotiated that will cover some evaluation, training, equipment, transportation and rehabilitation costs. In this respect, it is fiscally desirable to arrange an evaluation and training time for the homebound individual, to reach desired productivity levels. In view of the income needed by voluntary agencies from service fees, within the limits of reason and good rehabilitation agency practice, the longer the period of state rehabilitation agency sponsorship, the less will be the financial burden that ultimately falls upon the long-term service agency.

When service fees run out and the agency and the client stand fiscally naked and alone, reality begins to set in. In the first place, in having rehabilitated the homebound client under state rehabilitation agency auspices, the homebound service organization assumes an actual or implied responsibility to deliver long-term service to the individual in the post-rehabilitation period. In some instances, this responsibility can be diminished by placing the client with a private employer, obtaining the cooperation of one or more community agencies, or qualifying for workshop grants as offered now in a few states, through which state funds are paid annually to agencies providing long-term workshop (or homebound) service in stipulated situations.

In the long-run, however, post-rehabilitation homebound employment or services will have to be supported by self-sustaining income derived from work activities and from philanthropic contributions. In the former instance, exceptional management skill is needed to negotiate fair prices for contracts and materials and to maintain program expenses at a reasonable level, thus assuring the client a satisfactory income. No businessman in private industry is ever faced with a more demanding administrative situation. By definition, homebound manpower is limited manpower, and costly supportive services are essential. Expensive transportation is needed, and suitable work for the home is hard to come by. Thus, it is a tribute to sagacity, professional maturity, and talent of rehabilitation administrators that many of them are maintaining homebound rehabilitation programs at a solvent level. Some economies are possible through the recruitment and assignment of volunteers, the part-time use in homebound rehabilitation of staff members already engaged in other agency functions, combining the needs of homebound programming with other programming in scheduling transportation, obtaining family cooperation in the pickup and delivery of materials, and pooling contracts between the agency's sheltered workshop and homework programs so that each can supplement the other.

Although funding problems have to be faced, they are by no means insuperable. Thus, Federation of the Handicapped and more than thirty other voluntary agencies have undertaken continuing responsibility for the employment of homebound persons over long periods of time without experiencing overwhelming economic strain. Indeed, administrators of homebound rehabilitation programs are astute and prudent managers as well as visionary leaders. None of them could afford to retain their homebound service programs if, over the long-run, these programs so seriously depleted agency resources that service to other groups was being impaired.

Most homebound rehabilitation programs initiated thus far in the United States survive; sometimes their continuous history goes back more than a generation (Wisconsin Homecrafters and

Federation of the Handicapped). An examination of the stability of more recently developed programs suggests that few are experiencing serious financial trouble of such a character as to place the service in jeopardy.

The Administrator Looks Ahead

The Rehabilitation Act of 1973 emphasizes rehabilitation services for the severely disabled (including the homebound and the institutionalized). It is still too early to foresee the precise impact which this will have upon rehabilitation programming in the next five to ten years. However, a few predictions are possible at this time:

A. Building upon the impetus generated by the Programmatic Research Project on the Rehabilitation of Homebound Persons, the movement toward wider, more effective, and better supported homebound rehabilitation programs will accelerate in all parts of the United States.

B. Existing models will be used more extensively than ever as foundations for new programs while adventuresome agencies at the outer edge explore promising new leads and approaches that, in time, will become accepted rehabilitation practice.

C. Emerging advocacy programs will focus increasingly upon the severely disabled and, in the process, will call for strengthened homebound rehabilitation programs.

D. A growing number of cases in which rehabilitation services have been denied homebound persons will find their way into the courts and, as a result of the decisions reached in the judicial process, rehabilitation agencies will be mandated to serve homebound persons just as institutions now are being required by the courts to provide educational and rehabilitation services to their mentally retarded and emotionally disabled residents.

E. The mounting demand for more sophisticated homebound rehabilitation programs will sharpen the need for a national center (and, perhaps, concomitant regional ones, as well) that can perform the research, demonstration, and utilization activities that are needed to establish home-bound services on a more scientific basis.

F. Administrators, practitioners, family members, and community leaders will need extensive training in the concepts and techniques of rehabilitating homebound persons. Consequently, both short and long-term training programs will be established for this purpose.

G. Finally, and most important of all, a far larger proportion of the homebound people of America, currently neglected and exploited will be rehabilitated and will achieve a new and more functional status in our society and become taxpaying, contributing, and accepted members of their communities.

CHAPTER 14

VOCATIONAL HOMEMAKING AND INDEPENDENT LIVING IN THE REHABILITATION FACILITY

Lois O. Schwab

TODAY THERE ARE approximately ten million homemakers with physical disabilities. They represent the largest, single occupational group in the nation. About four million of these women have involvements due to cardiovascular disease; another three million have some form of arthritis. Hemiplegia, tuberculosis and orthopedic disabilities inflict the other three million women. These figures serve as a justification for rehabilitation programs in homemaking for women with physical disabilities.

Additionally, the number of women with mental health problems is increasing in the population. Approximately ten million persons are classified as having some form of mental illness with another 250,000 new patients undergoing treatment each year. Presumably, approximately half of these persons with mental illness are women.

Purpose of Program

A large percentage of the handicapped women presented in the above statistics have some housekeeping tasks and homemaking responsibilities. These women are in most respects no different from the so-called *normal* women. They have basic requirements, as other individuals, for satisfaction of physical needs, for security, for love and affection, and for being important to someone. Some or all of these requirements may be threatened by her disability. She may feel insecure, unloved, and unlovely because of society's ideal of physical perfection or in her limitation of performing the tasks required of women in the Western culture. Each of these women is faced with the challenge and the necessity of making adjustments in light of her handicapped condition, in her ways of functioning and/or her physical surroundings in order to meet her own and, in many cases, her family's needs. The problem of handicapped women takes on special importance because of the roles which women have in Western culture. The wife and mother occupies a keystone position in the family as she generally performs many routine jobs for and gives psychological support to each member of the family for activities inside and outside the home. Latest statistics show that 55 percent of married women between the ages of twenty-one to sixty-five years are not engaged in so-called gainful employment (work for pay inside or outside the home).

For many men and woman in the world of work, the occurrence of a handicapping condition is followed by retraining for a new job wherein maximum use can be made of limited body or mind. In the case of the handicapped homemaker, there usually is no new job outside the home for which she is to be trained. Her work remains in her home and her occupation continues to be that of homemaker.

Homemaking as a vocational role has a recognized monetary value. Recent studies place this value at between $5,000–$10,000 a year depending on family size (Walker and Gauger, 1973). Even the wife/mother with a small family and a part-time job outside the home spends a number of hours in household work in the home. Women with severe disabilities can and do continue their homemaking responsibilities. The following table gives

TABLE II

TIME SPENT IN HOMEMAKING TASKS BY HOMEMAKERS CONFINED TO WHEELCHAIRS AND VALUE OF HOMEMAKING TIME

N = 30

Tasks	Weekly Time Average Hours[1]	Minimum-Wage Dollar/Hr.[*]	Time-Value Dollars
Food-related activities	19.0	$2.27	$ 43.13
House care	7.7	2.00	15.40
Clothing and textile care	7.6	2.00	15.20
Physical care of others	1.9	2.00	3.80
Financial management and marketing	2.2	2.57	5.65
Total per week	38.4	——	$ 83.18
Total per year	1,996.8	——	$4,325.36

[1] M. Merchant, *Homemaking Time Use of Homemakers Confined to Wheelchairs.* Unpublished M.S. thesis, University of Nebraska, 1969.

[*] Minimum entry rate for institutions in Nebraska Personnel System.

monetary value to selected time expenditures of severely disabled homemakers confined to the wheelchair. Individuals with lesser handicaps might well be spending more time in household work. Additionally, it is recognized that most women are more skilled and hence, worth more per hour than a minimum wage represents.

Independent Living for All Handicapped

All individuals, men, women and children, have the right to a training whereby they can reach optimum levels for "doing for themselves," in such activities as dressing, toileting, eating and even preparing their own food. Educational programs for handicapped persons of all ages, children through the aged, should include these facets not only because of the self-respect which comes from "doing it myself" but also because of the high costs of any form of assistance or custodial care.

Governmental agencies at all levels recognize that the alternatives of institutionalization and provision of personal services are costly. The third route of helping individuals is attractive because it emphasizes independence with the individuals still "in charge" of themselves. The skills developed for the sustaining of self are usually those which are transferable to "workbench" and office for gainful employment. Individuals with handicaps must be helped to attain self-maintenance.

All children with physical handicaps, all men and women with physical handicaps of the working age as well as the elderly with major physical impairments (totaling 30 million persons) should benefit from basic instruction in independent living.

Homemaking Rehabilitation Center for
the Physically Disabled

Generally, the problems of homemakers focus on two main aspects; these are (1) limitations in the functioning of the body as with paralysis, amputation, or impaired functioning of the arm, or low energy level, and (2) physical obstacles in the near environment, such as steps which cannot be climbed in a wheelchair, and cupboards which cannot be reached from a seated position.

A comprehensive rehabilitation center should offer laboratory space for the women/men with various physical disabilities to try out for themselves the kinds of adjustments in the near environment which are proposed for them. Generally, the laboratory should include two kitchens. One should have normal thirty-six inch high counters and standard equipment for the ambulatory disabled (those who use canes, walkers, crutches or who may *not* use any devices), and one should have counters and cupboards adjusted for work from wheelchair or other chair. Laboratory space should also demonstrate adjustments possible in the laundry center, bedroom and bathroom.

Physical handicaps come in various types and degrees for individuals of all types and of both sexes so planning and adjustments for a particular home becomes an individual affair. A laboratory area should be designed so that as many adjustments as possible may be tried by the various clients of an agency. A few generalizations explain the problem. The standard wheelchair decreases a person's height by one-third and doubles his width. A pathway of at least five feet by five feet of clear area is needed for turnabout of a wheelchair. These statistics will change with use of the junior size wheelchair or the chair on a motorized platform with wheels and a steering handle. Dimensions for homes for two persons with the same disability might be quite different due to body measurements, choice and use of mobility device, and degree of independence desired.

Kitchen for Chair-Confined Persons

The kitchen should have a mix center, a sink area and a cooking-baking area. A number of arrangements of these areas is possible and may work for a particular individual, but the L-arrangement accommodates the wheelchair-confined person allowing at least four feet in front of each area for moving of wheelchair. It gives the needed room for the maneuvering of the wheelchair and for accommodation of an assistant also working in the kitchen. New standardized factory-built cupboards and cabinets (30 inches without counter) in module units can be purchased for laboratory use.

Generally, the mix center should be twenty-seven to thirty-two inches high with a desk-type counter.* The space below the counter for the knees should be at least twenty-eight inches wide. Another work height for other jobs to be done in this area is recommended; this can best be obtained through use of a pull-out work board twenty-four to twenty-nine inches from the floor.

The sink should be shallow with a four and one-half to five inches depth. To accommodate the sink depth, this counter may best be placed at twenty-nine to thirty-three inches from the floor. Again, individual measurements, such as kind of chair and thickness of thigh, become additional factors in determining this height. The desk-type opening for this center should be at least twenty-eight inches wide and have insulation at top and back to protect thighs and knees from hot water in pipes and bowl.

The oven should be low enough for the homemaker using it to remove dishes easily. Generally, the lower shelf is placed thirty-two inches from the floor. An oven with a side-opening door is advisable; the door should open to give easy access to the nearby work counter.

Kitchen for General Use

The traditional kitchen has all work counters at a standardized height of thirty-six inches from the floor. It is to be recognized that neither man nor woman has been bred to this standard size. Kitchen work areas should allow for the testing of proper height for a person through use of an adjustable height counter. Persons of four feet eight inches height and six feet four inches are both handicapped when trying to use the customary thirty-six inch counter. The adjustable work area for trial purposes should have a range of twenty-eight to forty-two inches from the floor.

A kitchen should have some general functional features; these apply to the kitchen for the chair-confined as well as the normal, healthy person:

---

* It is recognized that many individuals with limited energy and/or ambulatory problems find it easier to sit down to work at any job that takes more than a few minutes.

a. Counters at least fifteen inches wide should be built next to the oven, range units and refrigerator for placing dishes.
b. The refrigerator and freezer compartment with easily-opened doors should be placed as near as possible to the sink and range centers to eliminate excessive travel.
c. A wheeled table eliminates steps when transporting food and dishes to and from the dining area.
d. Appropriate energy-saving equipment should be included: dishwasher, electric disposal, electric mixer, range surface units, oven or portable combination oven-broiler. Other equipment such as a blender, garbage compactor, may be advantageous to certain persons.

Other Considerations for Homemaking Center for the Physically Disabled

Programs in homemaking and/or independent living for individuals with physical disabilities should have laboratory space which has been adjusted to the special needs of individuals with any of a broad range of physical limitations. Adjustments for those in wheelchairs are of special concern and are listed below. The following specifications do not apply to centers for the emotionally disturbed but some ideas may be incorporated as a matter of safety.

Laundry Center

The laundry (Kehm and Schwab, 1973) area should be conveniently located on the main floor at a point where there is the most laundry.

Front-loading washers and dryers with easily-reached controls are best for the persons confined to wheelchairs. The top-loading washers and dryers are most convenient for those using crutches or walkers.

A table for sorting and/or folding laundry should be available next to either washer/dryer or both at a height usable to the seated person. Because ironing boards come in an assortment of types and sizes, considerable attention should be given to an adjustable height which allows for working while seated. The kind of lifting required for placing many of the boards up and down may be too much for many individuals. A wall-hung closet with adjustable ironing board is available. Racks and tables should be allowed adjacent to the board for baskets of unironed linens and clothing as well as for the ironed clothing and flat linens.

A laundry cart and convenient storage space should be included.

Bedroom

The bed should be accessible by wheelchair with at least three feet of clearance on both sides and around the foot of the bed. The mattress should be approximately nineteen inches from the floor in order to be level with the seat of the wheelchair for those who are chair-confined. A light switch, preferably a master switch for the house, should be within easy reach of the person while in bed. There should also be a pushbutton near the head of the bed for activating an audio and visual alarm unit located outside the housing unit.

A closet should be easily available with either sliding or outswinging half doors. One rod should be no higher than forty-eight inches from the floor. The dressing table should be thirty to thirty-two inches high with a desk-type opening with a width of twenty-eight inches.

Bathroom

A bathroom should be adjacent to the bedroom of the person with physical limitation. Again, as with other parts of the center, all details must be considered to make possible independence in this area.

The toilet seat should be higher than the usual chair for most individuals. A nineteen inch high seat is recommended; this is to be gained through an elevated seat three to four inches high, a wooden platform under the standard toilet stool, or a wall-hung stool located higher on the wall. Horizontal grab bars at thirty-three inches from floor should be available. The mounting of the lavatory is important. The individual's own measurements and the type of wheelchair are usually most important considerations (although it may range from 28-34 inches). However, a height of thirty-two inches from the floor is recommended for the lavatory counter. Often, a round eighteen inch in diameter lavatory with mixer faucets and wand control is mounted sideways to make for easy reach by the person seated on the toilet stool. Mirrors should be lowered so the bottom edge begins at forty inches from the floor. Soap dishes and towel racks should be reachable.

A bathroom door should have locks which are functional from either side. Again, a pushbutton for activating an alarm with audio and visual signal outside the living unit should be reachable from either tub or toilet. Adequate storage for linens and personal supplies should be available in the toilet area.

A tub should have a number of features for safety and ease; these include an abrasive, non-slip bottom, a substantial bench for sitting at a higher height for those who find it difficult to lower or raise themselves from a floor position, and water controls, preferably a mixing faucet, with non-scald temperature control, accessible from the bathing position.

A shower should have a stall doorway with at least a clear opening of thirty-two inches, a slightly sloping floor which starts level with room floor without obstructing riser or curb, floor with a non-slip surface, handrail at least on one side to facilitate going in and out, a seat with a smooth, easily-cleaned surface, and a mixing faucet with non-scald temperature control.

Other General Recommendations for the Rehabilitation Center

Floors should have a nonslip surface. If carpets are used, they should have a firm tuft for easy maneuvering because deep shag carpeting often makes it difficult to guide a wheelchair. Small scatter rugs should be eliminated.

Light switches should be aligned with door handles at thirty-six inches from the floor. Electric outlets should not be placed lower than two feet above the floor.

A telephone should be available near the center of house, if only one is available, at a height no higher than forty-eight inches.

Doors should have clear, unobstructed opening at least thirty-two inches wide; lever-type handles, and thresholds flush with floor or less than one-half inch high.

Windows should have easy-to-operate, easy-to-reach mechanisms, such as bar or gear-type handles and have panes beginning no higher than thirty-six inches above floor level.

For a home checklist, see *Barrier-free Housing* in *1973 Yearbook of Agriculture* entitled Handbook for Home.

Personnel for Program

Home economists have considered improved home and family living as the central focus of their profession. Rehabilitation programs become a natural component of this focus. Rehabilitation personnel teaching homemaking and independent living should have competencies in each area of home economics as well as an expertise in rehabilitation counseling. In a recent study by Knoll and Schwab (1974) more than 33 percent of the 255 rehabilitation administrators recommended that the home economist have coursework emphasizing counseling techniques and psychological aspects of the disability. Home economists desiring to work with the physically handicapped should also have coursework in medical aspects of physical disability. Furthermore, 64 percent of the administrators of programs for the emotionally disturbed reported a willingness to add a home economist to the staff, and 74 percent of the administrators of programs for the physically disabled would like a home economist added to the staff. Of these administrators, 22 percent were making actual plans to add the home economist to their staff. These administrators generally recognize that additional coursework beyond the bachelor's degree in home economics would be needed.

According to Fadul (1973), seven home economics units in higher education have offered the opportunity for specialization in the rehabilitation field. These units are located at:

Colorado State University
University of Georgia
Southern Illinois University
University of Missouri
University of Nebraska-Lincoln

Ohio State University, Columbus, Ohio

Pennsylvania State University, University Park, Pennsylvania

In many instances, occupational therapists are also being prepared for helping clients in the areas of homemaking and independent living. Not all programs include these facets, but occupational therapists may attend short courses and workshops being conducted to add this dimension to their expertise.

Records and Reports

Evaluation of each client's ability in performing tasks and functioning as an individual should be recorded as a basis for a rehabilitation program. These become the records on which judgments are made. For the various types of programs with the physically disabled at the University of Nebraska-Lincoln, the following forms have been used:

INTERVIEW FOR HOMEMAKER EVALUATION

(Physical Disability)

Statement of disability: ....

Length of time since onset: ....

Appliances used: Wheelchair ......; Crutch(es) L ...... R ......;
               Brace(s) L ...... R ......; Cane(s) L...... R......;
               Walker ....

Sitting position: Good ......; Difficult ......; Poor ....
               Comments: ....

Handedness: Dominant hand R ...... L ......
           One hand only R ...... L ......

Problems: Weakness .... Fatigue ....

          Incoordination .... Vision ....

          Spasticity .... Hearing ....

          Pain .... Speech ....

          Fear of failure .... Intellectual ....

Involvement of:

Arms	R		Shoulders	R ......
	L			L ......
Hands	R		Hip(s)	R ......
	L			L ......
Fingers	R		Leg(s)	R ......
	L			L ......
Wrists	R		Feet	R ......
	L			L ......
Elbows	R		Ankles	R ......
	L			L ......
Upper Trunk	....		Knees	R ......
				L ......

Other: ....

INTERVIEW FOR HOMEMAKER EVALUATION

(Homemaker Activities and Family Attitude)

Information to be indirectly ascertained.
Indicate the activities that are difficult or tiring for the homemaker.
Bending forward at the hips ....
What jobs require bending? ....
Bending at the knees to stoop ....
Where do you do this in your daily activities? ....
....
Reaching ....
Where do you have to reach or stretch? ....
....
Climbing (stairs or to reach high storage) ....
Where must you climb? ....
Lifting ....
Where must you lift? ....
Carrying ....
What must you carry and how far? ....
Standing ....
For what jobs must you stand long enough to get tired? ....
....
Walking ....
Where must you walk a great deal? ....
General impressions (observations by researcher):
Adeptness in homemaking ....
....
....
Attitude toward homemaking ....
....
Family attitude toward patient's role as homemaker ....
....
....

INTERVIEW FOR HOMEMAKER EVALUATION

(Homemaking and the Family)

Information to be indirectly ascertained.
Homemaker's stated problems: ....
....
....
Homemaker's activities:
What activities do you perform most successfully? ....
....
What adjustments have been made to make this possible? ....
....
What activities are most difficult for you? ....
....
Why? ....

Satisfactions in homemaking:
Which homemaking jobs are most important for *you* to do? . . . .
. . . .
What jobs of homemaking give you the most satisfaction? . . . .
. . . .
Responsibility:
How much responsibility should children assume? . . . .
. . . .
Do your children have more or less responsibility than you desire? . . . .
What do your children do to help? . . . .
. . . .
Does your husband help at home? . . . .
What jobs does he do? . . . .
Do you wish he would do more or less? . . . .
Does he do more or less than other husbands? . . . .
Is he a "handyman" for making changes? . . . .
Recreation:
What kind of outside activities are your children engaged in? . . . .
. . . .
Are you able to spend as much time as you would like with your husband and
children? . . . .
. . . .
Have there been changes in your relationship with your children since you
have become disabled? . . . .
If so, what changes? . . . .
. . . .
What kinds of things do you do for pleasure? . . . .
. . . .
What do you and your husband do together? . . . .
. . . .
In what activities did you participate before your disability? . . . .
. . . .
Assistance:
Who has helped you in any way since you became disabled? . . . .
. . . .
What agencies have helped you? . . . .
. . . .
What help have you wanted and not received? . . . .
. . . .
Perceived objectives of training: . . . .
. . . .
. . . .
. . . .
. . . .
. . . .
. . . .
. . . .
. . . .

INDIVIDUAL MEASUREMENTS

Height when standing _____ Date _____

Height when seated _____

Height for chair-seat _____

Height of chair-arm _____

desk-type __ yes __ no __

Use only appropriate measurements:

	Standing	Stool	Chair	Wheel-chair
Maximum depth reach at counter				
Maximum useful reach when arms extended (90°)				
Height of elbows — (arms close to body)				
Maximum useful height with lap under counter				
Normal easy reach below counter (135°)				
Maximum reach below counter				
Maximum reach to low storage with lap under counter				
Most comfortable height for:				
Ironing				
Dishwashing (bottom of sink)				
Mixing-Handheld electric mixer				

INDIVIDUAL MEASUREMENTS – – Continued

	Standing	Stool	Chair	Wheel-chair
Hand-held rotary beater				
Wooden spoon – in bowl				
Rolling Pastry				
Chopping vegetable				

Note:

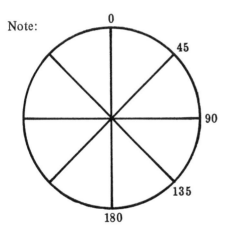

Degrees of Reach

Cooperating Agencies

In each state there are different groups of agencies who have an interest in the area of homemaking rehabilitation and independent living. These may vary from such groups as the State-Federal Cooperative Extension Service to the Visiting Nurses. Each community is different.

State-Federal Cooperative Extension Service

Across the nation, home economists of the United States Department of Agriculture have realized that the dimension of help to the physically and mentally handicapped should be added to their educational services. Presently, seventeen states have included some program emphasis. Home economists in these states are available for individual and group consultation in regard to both homemaking and independent living consideration.

State-Federal Rehabilitation Services Administration

The state-federal rehabilitation agencies are now showing approximately one-sixth of the closures of clients in the homemaking category. Because of this, home economists trained in rehabilitation counseling are being brought onto the staffs of these rehabilitation agencies to conduct work with individuals with physical and/or mental handicaps. These programs may emphasize training with a minimum of remodeling of homes. The cooperative program of the Nebraska Division of Rehabilitation Services and the University of Nebraska-Lincoln has been able to provide appropriate training averaging less than $300 per client.

Conclusion

The inclusion of the homemaking component in the comprehensive rehabilitation center not only serves more than half of the women clients but also many of the men. This service under properly trained personnel will not only serve as a retraining area for women clients in a vocational role but also means a training in independent living for men, children, and youth.

The training in self-care and care of home includes gaining many skills which are transferable to workbench and office.

REFERENCES

Fadul, R.: Home Economics and Rehabilitation in Institutions of Higher Education. Unpublished master's thesis, University of Nebraska-Lincoln, 1973.

Kehm, V., and Schwab, L.: *Laundry Equipment and Arrangements for Chair-Confined Homemakers.* Department of Education and Family Resources Report No. 1. Lincoln, University of Nebraska, 1973.

Knoll, C., and Schwab, L.: The outlook for home economists in rehabilitation. *Journal of Home Economics, 66:*39-42, 1974.

Merchant, M.: Homemaking Time Use of Homemakers Confined to Wheelchairs. Unpublished master's thesis, University of Nebraska-Lincoln, 1969.

Schwab, L.: Barrier-free housing for the handicapped. In *Handbook for the Home, the 1973 Yearbook of Agriculture.* Washington, D. C., United States Department of Agriculture, 1973, pp. 228-235.

Walker, K., and Gauger, W.: *The Dollar Value of Household Work.* Ithaca, New York College of Human Ecology, 1973.

INDEX